CHRISTIAN HENDRICH, ULRICH NÖTH, JOCHEN EULERT (Eds.)

Cartilage Surgery and Future Perspectives

D1726989

Springer

Berlin
Heidelberg
New York
Hong Kong
London
Milan
Paris
Tokyo

Christian Hendrich, Ulrich Nöth,
Jochen Eulert (Eds.)

Cartilage Surgery and Future Perspectives

With 109 Figures and 14 Tables

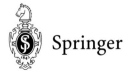 Springer

CHRISTIAN HENDRICH, M.D.
Associate Professor
Orthopaedic Institute
König-Ludwig-Haus
Julius-Maximilians-University
Würzburg, Germany

ULRICH NÖTH, M.D.
Head, Division of Tissue Engineering
Orthopaedic Institute
König-Ludwig-Haus
Julius-Maximilians-University
Würzburg, Germany

JOCHEN EULERT, M.D.
Professor and Chairman
Orthopaedic Institute
König-Ludwig-Haus
Julius-Maximilians-University
Würzburg, Germany

ISBN 3-540-01054-8   Springer-Verlag Berlin Heidelberg New York
Cataloging-in-Publication Date applied for
Cartilage Surgery and Future Perspectives, C. Hendrich, U. Nöth, J. Eulert - Berlin;
Heidelberg; New York; Hong Kong; London; Milan; Paris; Tokyo; Springer, 2003
    ISBN 3-540-01054-8

Springer-Verlag is a company in the BertelsmannSpringer Publishing Group
© Springer-Verlag Berlin Heidelberg 2003
Printed in Germany

Product liability: The publisher cannot guarantee the accuracy of any information
about dosage and application contained in this book. In every individual case the user
must check such information by consulting the relevant literature.

Cover-Design: design & production GmbH, Heidelberg
Typesetting: TypoStudio Tobias Schaedla, Heidelberg

Printed on acid-free paper –   SPIN 109 10 894   18/5141 – 5 4 3 2 1 0 –

Foreword

Tissue engineering as a technology and as a therapeutic has captured worldwide attention and commitment because it has such potential in the care of humanity. Because we are not as yet able to craft robust three-dimensional vascular and ductal structures to support the development of complex parenchymal organs, the initial focus of the field has been on thin tissues that can be nourished by diffusion alone. The best example of this class is cartilage.

Thought by some to be a relatively simple tissue in the early days of tissue engineering, deep study of this tissue has shown it to manifest great complexity. Years of experimental and clinical effort have begun to untangle the clues that will allow us to reproducibly characterize, generate and clinically apply engineered cartilage with positive effects. Worldwide researchers and clinicians are intently focused on this goal and it has come time to step back and make a good assessment of our progress.

The Editors, Christian Hendrich, Ulrich Nöth and Jochen Eulert have provided us with a volume that is designed to do just that. It is a pleasure to see that they have designed their book to provide an overview of the field as a whole, provided a primer on cartilage biology, a review of the raw materials that have classically been used in the design of engineered cartilage and have stressed the emerging role of mesenchymal stem cell science in cartilage repair. This will make the book highly accessible to the general clinical and scientific readership, since all elements, including the clinical experience, have been placed into context. They have also astutely provided us with a vision for future development of the field.

We are fortunate to have this update on cartilage tissue engineering. The efforts of the authors and editors merit our thanks.

Peter C. Johnson, M.D.
Chairman and CEO, TissueInformatics Inc.
Immediate Past President, Tissue Engineering Society International
pcj@tissueinformatics.com; www.tissueinformatics.com

Preface

For more than two centuries, since Hunter in 1743, damaged articular cartilage was thought to be irreparable. Today, there are a number of treatment strategies in clinical use. These include a simple lavage and debridement, abrasion, drilling, microfracturing, transplantation of osteochondral auto- or allografts, and the autologous chondrocyte transplantation (ACT). Brittberg and Peterson published first clinical results of the ACT in 1994. This work was the beginning of a new era employing cell-based technology for articular cartilage repair. Together with the rapidly growing field of tissue engineering, new technologies in scaffold processing and stem cell biology many promising experimental strategies using different scaffold materials and cell sources have been developed. This book gives an overview of the outcome of surgical techniques currently in clinical use and new promising approaches for future articular cartilage repair. Special thanks goes to all contributors for sharing with us their experience and expertise making it possible to give a state of the art overview of "Cartilage Surgery and Future Perspectives". Also, we want to thank the industry for their generous support, Thomas Günther from Springer-Verlag, Heidelberg, for the enthusiasm he put in publishing this book and all research funding institutions.

Würzburg, April 2003

The editors
CHRISTIAN HENDRICH
ULRICH NÖTH
JOCHEN EULERT

Table of Contents

List of Editors

CHRISTIAN HENDRICH, M.D.
Associate Professor
Orthopaedic Institute
König-Ludwig-Haus
Julius-Maximilians-University
Würzburg, Germany

ULRICH NÖTH, M.D.
Head, Division of Tissue Engineering
Orthopaedic Institute
König-Ludwig-Haus
Julius-Maximilians-University
Würzburg, Germany

JOCHEN EULERT, M.D.
Professor and Chairman
Orthopaedic Institute
König-Ludwig-Haus
Julius-Maximilians-University
Würzburg, Germany

List of First Authors

WILHELM K. AICHER, PH.D.
Basic Science Research Laboratory
Center of Orthopaedic Surgery
Eberhard-Karls-University
Tübingen, Germany

THOMAS AIGNER, M.D.
Cartilage Research
Department of Pathology
Erlangen-Nürnberg-University
Erlangen, Germany

ERHAN BASAD, M.D.
Department of Orthopaedic Surgery
Justus-Liebig-University
Gießen, Germany

ACHIM BATTMANN, M.D.
Institute of Pathology
Justus-Liebig-University
Gießen, Germany

JOACHIM GRIFKA, M.D.
Professor and Chairman
Department of Orthopaedic Surgery
University of Regensburg
Bad Abbach, Germany

CHRISTIAN HENDRICH, M.D.
Associate Professor
Orthopaedic Institute
König-Ludwig-Haus
Julius-Maximilians-University
Würzburg, Germany

HARTMUT F. HILDEBRAND, PH.D.
Professor/INSERM Research Director
Head, Laboratory of Biomaterial Research
Faculty of Medicine
Lille-Cedex, France

PETER C. JOHNSON, M.D.
Chairman and Chief Executive Officer
Tissue Informatics. Inc
Pittsburgh, PA, USA

ULRICH NÖTH, M.D.
Head, Division of Tissue Engineering
Orthopaedic Institute
König-Ludwig-Haus
Julius-Maximilians-University
Würzburg, Germany

CARSTEN PERKA, M.D.
Associate Professor
Department of Orthopaedics
Charité-University Hospital
Berlin, Germany

LARS PETERSON, M.D., PH.D.
Professor, Department of Orthopaedics
Sahlgrenska University Hospital
University of Gothenburg and
Clinical Director
Gothenburg Medical Center
Västra Frölunda, Sweden

HANS PISTNER, M.D., D.D.S., PH.D.
Associate Professor and Chairman
Department of Cranio-Maxillo-Facial and Regional Plastic Surgery
HELIOS-Klinikum
Erfurt, Germany

BRIGITTE VON RECHENBERG, M.D., DVN
Associate Professor
Dipl. ECVS
Musculoskeletal Research Unit
Equine Hospital, Faculty of Veternary Medicine
University of Zürich
Zürich, Switzerland

MAXIMILIAN RUDERT, M.D.
Associate Professor
Department of Orthopaedic Surgery
Eberhard-Karls-University
Tübingen, Germany

ULRICH SCHNEIDER, M.D.
Associate Professor
Department of Orthopaedic Surgery
RWTH-University Hospital
Aachen, Germany

MICHAEL SITTINGER, PH.D.
Associate Professor
Tissue Engineering Laboratories
Department of Rheumatology and Clinical Immunology
Berlin Medical Faculty Charité
Berlin, Germany

MATTHIAS STEINWACHS, M.D.
Head, Cartilage Research Group
Valley Tissue Engineering Center Freiburg
Clinic for Orthopaedic Surgery
Department of Orthopaedics und Trauma Surgery
Albert-Ludwigs-University
Freiburg, Germany

ROCKY S.TUAN, PH.D.
Professor and Branch Chief
Cartilage Biology and Orthopaedics Branch
National Institute of Arthritis, Muscoloskeletal & Skin Diseases (NIAMS)
National Institutes of Health (NIH)
Bethesda, MD, USA

ANDREAS WERNER, M.D.
Associate Professor
Department of Orthopaedic Surgery
Heinrich-Heine-University
Düsseldorf, Germany

ULRICH ZIMMERMANN, PH.D.
Professor and Chairman
Department of Biotechnology
Julius-Maximilians-University
Würzburg, Germany

List of Abbreviations

ACI	autologous chondrocyte implantation
ACL	anterior cruciate ligament
ACT	autologous chondrocyte transplantation
ADAMTS	a disintegrin and metalloproteinase with thrombospondin type motif 1
AFM	atomic force microscopy
ALK-1	activin-like kinase 1
AOTAS	American Orthopaedic Foot and Ankle Society
AP	alkaline phosphatase
ASTM	American Society for Testing and Materials
bFGF	basic fibroblast growth factor
BMI	body mass index
BMP	bone morphogenetic protein
CD	cluster of differentiation
CFU	colony forming unit
CFU-F	colony forming unit fibroblast
CLIP	cartilage intermediate layer protein
CG	clinical grade
CLSM	confocal laser scanning microscopy
COMP	cartilage oligomeric protein
CPM	continuous passive motion
CTGF	connective tissue growth factor
DAB	diaminobenzidine
DGKKT	Deutsche Gesellschaft für autologe Knorpel- und Knochenzelltransplantation
DGOOC	Deutsche Gesellschaft für Orthopädie und Orthopädische Chirurgie
DGU	Deutsche Gesellschaft für Unfallchirurgie
DMEM	Dulbecco's Modified Eagle's Medium
DMSO	dimethyl sulfoxide
ECM	extracellular matrix
EDTA	ethylene-diamine-tetra-acetic acid
EGF	epidermal growth factor
FC	femoral condyle
FCS	fetal calf serum

FGF	fibroblast growth factor
FPCL	fibroblast populated collagen lattice
GAGs	glycoseaminoglycans
GAPDH	glyceraldehyde-3-phosphatase dehydrogenase
GDF	growth differentiation factor
GMP	good manufacturing practice
HA	hyaluronic acid
HE	haematoxylin eosin
HSA	human serum albumin
HSS	Hospital for Special Surgery
ICRS	International Cartilage Repair Society
IKDC	International Knee Documentation Committee
IL	interleukin
ISO	International Standardization Organization
MACI	matrix-induced autologous chondrocyte implantation
MCP	metacarpophalangeal
MG	Masson-Goldner
MMP	matrix metalloproteinase
mRNA	messenger RNA
MSC	mesenchymal stem cell
N	Newton
NMR	nuclear magnetic resonance
OCD	osteochondritis dissecans
OCT	osteochondral transplantation
PAP	peroxidase-antiperoxidase technique
PCR	polymerase chain reaction
PDGF	platelet-derived growth factor
PGA	polyglycolic acid
PIC	polyion complex
PLA	polylactic acid
PLLA	poly-L-lactic acid
qRT-PCR	quantitative reverse transcription polymerase chain reaction
RNA	ribonucleic acid
ROM	range of motion
RT	real-time
SD	standard deviation
SEM	scanning electron microscopy
Smad	small body size mother against decapentaplegic
TCP	tricalcium phosphate
TGF	transforming growth factor
TNFα	tumor necrosis factor α
UHV-CG	ultra-high viscosity clinical-grade
VAS	visual analog scale

Basics

I

Anatomy and Biochemistry of Articular Cartilage*

1

Thomas Aigner and Zhiyong Fan

Articular cartilage is a highly specialized and uniquely designed biomaterial that forms the smooth and gliding surface of diarthrodial joints. It is an avascular, aneural and alymphatic matrix, which is synthesized by the sparsely distributed resident cells – the chondrocytes, which are considered to be largely postmitotic cells in the adult [12]. The functional element, as in all connective tissues, is clearly the extracellular matrix, which enables the painless movement over the lifespan (Fig. 1.1). The cells are the viable elements of articular cartilage and are responsible for the maintenance of the extracellular matrix.

Morphology of Articular Cartilage

The adult hyaline articular cartilage, which forms the surface of articulating joints, can essentially be divided into four separate zones: the superficial, the middle, the deep, and the calcified zone (Fig. 1.2) [14]. Besides the integrity of the cartilage matrix, a smooth articular surface is crucial for the frictionless gliding of the articular surfaces during joint movement. In adult articular cartilage, cells of the superficial zone are small and flat and are oriented with the collagen fibers. In contrast, chondrocytes of the middle zone appear larger and more round with an apparent randomly distribution within the matrix. Also, the direction of the collagen fibers is more randomly structured. In the deeper zone, the cells form columns lying perpendicular to the cartilage surface, as do the collagen fibers. The lowest zone is calcified and close to the subchondral bone plate. The zone seems to form an intermediate layer between the elastic cartilage and the stiff bone. Cells in this zone are to a large portion dead or vanished [1]. Interestingly, the chondrocytes themselves appear to behave different depending on their position within the different layers of the cartilage matrix [3, 4]. Thus, the cells of the middle and deep zone appear to be most metabolic active.

* This work was supported by the Bundesministerium für Bildung und Forschung (BMBF; Grant # 01GG9824).

extracellular matrix =
functional element

articular
cartilage

chondrocyte =
reactive element

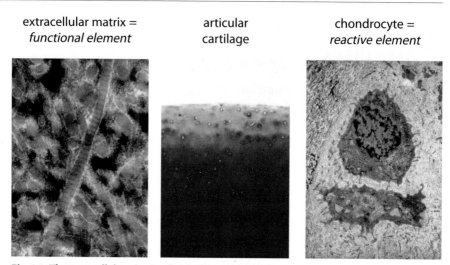

Fig. 1.1. The extracellular matrix of articular cartilage (electron micrograph on the left) represents the "functional element" (i.e. the essential component providing its biomechanic properties). The cells of the tissue (i.e. the chondrocytes: electron micrograph on the right) represent the active players, which synthesize most of the matrix degrading proteases and fully provide anabolic activity. The picture in the middle shows the normal histological appearance of articular cartilage.

superficial zone

middle

deep

calcified

bone

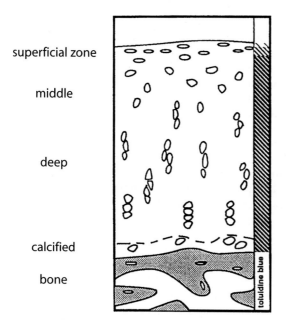

Fig. 1.2.
Zonal architecture of normal adult human articular cartilage consisting of the superficial, middle (= transitional), deep (= radial), and calcified zone.

Biochemistry of Articular Cartilage

At the supramolecular level the cartilage matrix consists of two basic components: a fibrillar and an extrafibrillar matrix. The fibrillar matrix is a network consisting mainly of type II and other collagens, predominantly types IX and XI [7]. The non-fibrillar component consists predominantly of highly sulfated aggrecan monomers, attached to hyaluronic acid and link protein, forming very large polyanionic aggregates. In terms of the physical properties of the matrix, tensile strength comes from the collagen network, which hinders expansion of the visco-elastic aggrecan component, providing compressive stiffness [10]. Under compressive force, the cartilage matrix is compliant and recovers rapidly its elasticity, as water is drawn back into the matrix by the hydrophilic aggrecan aggregates [9]. Cartilage matrix also contains a large number of other components that are important for matrix cohesion and for regulation of chondrocyte function. The small non-aggregating proteoglycans decorin, biglycan, and fibromodulin have all been detected in the extracellular matrix. There is evidence that decorin and fibromodulin may be involved in regulation of fibrillogenesis and growth factor binding. The role of biglycan has yet to be determined. Other matrix proteins that have been detected in the extracellular matrix include fibronectin, cartilage matrix protein and cartilage oligomeric protein (COMP), which may be involved in regulation of gene expression and the chondrogenic phenotype.

So far, most investigators have analyzed the pathobiochemistry of the interterritorial cartilage matrix. Much less attention has been paid to the pericellular cartilage matrix. At present, only collagen type VI has been well investigated. Collagen type VI is concentrated in the pericellular matrix in articular cartilage [13]. Ultra-structural studies have shown a physical overlap of the collagen type VI network with the type II positive matrix. This supports the notion that collagen type VI is a central molecular component forming a mechanical interface between the rigid type II matrix and the "soft" cell [15]. Other functions might include storage of growth factors and cell-matrix interaction.

Normal Turnover of the Extracellular Matrix

In normal human articular cartilage aggrecan and link protein are existing as heterogeneous populations, differing in size and composition, as a result of differential post-translational glycosylation and proteolysis [8]. Normal proteolytic aggrecan turnover is highly regulated and is most probably implemented by the action of matrix metalloproteinases (MMPs), particularly MMP-3. However, a second cleavage site, the "aggrecanase-site", has also been described in the interglobular domain and contributes to the proteolytic cleavage of aggrecan [2]. In normal adult articular cartilage the turnover of aggrecan is not excessive and the half-life of aggrecan monomers and aggregates depends very much on the matrix compartment, looking at ranges from days to months. Subdomains of the aggrecan core protein have even been measured to persist for years [11].

The collagen type II network is extremely stable. The tightly wound triple helices that constitute the collagen fibers are further stabilized by a high-degree of cross-link-

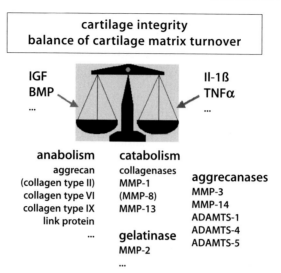

Fig. 1.3. The integrity of articular cartilage depends largely on a balance in cartilage matrix turnover. Listed are the major anabolic and catabolic gene products of human adult articular chondrocytes, as well as the most important anabolic and catabolic mediators of chondrocyte activity.

ing, which steadily increases with age [5]. Fiber destabilization can only be brought about by cleavage of the triple helix due to the action of collagenases, the most likely candidates for collagen type II being MMP-1 and MMP-13 [6]. Largely unknown are the turnover rates of the other molecular components of articular cartilage such as cartilage intermediate layer protein (CILP) and COMP. The matrix turnover, both anabolic and catabolic, is provided by the chondrocytes, which are stimulated by extracellular cytokines and growth factors (Fig. 1.3) and express matrix components as well as their degrading enzymes.

References

1. Aigner T, Hemmel M, Neureiter D, Gebhard PM, Zeiler G, Kirchner T et al. (2001) Apoptotic cell death is not a widespread phenomenon in normal aging and osteoarthritic human articular knee cartilage: A study of proliferation, programmed cell death (apoptosis), and viability of chondrocytes in normal and osteoarthritic human knee cartilage. Arthritis Rheum 44:1304–1312
2. Arner EC, Pratta MA, Tzaskos JM, Decicco CP, Tortorella MD (1999) Generation and characterization of aggrecanase. J Biol Chem 274:6594–6601
3. Aydelotte MB, Kuettner KE (1988) Differences between sub-populations of cultured bovine articular chondrocytes. I. Morphology and cartilage matrix production. Connect Tissue Res 18:205–222

4. Aydelotte MB, Greenhill RR, Kuettner KE (1988) Differences between sub-populations of cultured bovine articular chondrocytes. II. Proteoglycan metabolism. Connect Tissue Res 18:223–234

5. Bank RA, Bayliss MT, Lafeber FPJG, Maroudas A, TeKoppele JM (1997) Ageing and zonal variation in posttranslational modification of collagen in normal human articular cartilage. Biochem J 330:345–351

6. Billinghurst RC, Dahlberg L, Ionescu M, Reiner A, Bourne A, Rorabeck C et al. (1997) Enhanced cleavage of type II collagen by collagenase in osteoarthritic articular cartilage. J Clin Invest 99:1534–1545

7. Bruckner P, van der Rest M (1994) Structure and function of cartilage collagens. Microscop Res Tech 28:378–84

8. Buckwalter JA, Roughley PJ, Rosenberg LC (1994) Age-related changes in cartilage proteoglycans: quantitative electron microscopic studies. Microscop Res Tech 28:398–408

9. Carney SL, Muir H (1988) The structure and function of cartilage proteoglycans. Physiol Rev 68:858–910

10. Maroudas A (1976) Balance between swelling pressure and collagen tension in normal and degenerate cartilage. Nature 260:808–809

11. Maroudas A, Bayliss MT, Uchitel-Kaushansky N, Schneiderman R, Gilav E (1998) Aggrecan turnover in human articular cartilage: use of aspartic acid racemization as a marker of molecular age. Arch Biochem Biophys 350:61–71

12. Muir H (1995) The chondrocyte, architect of cartilage. BioEssays 17:1039–1048

13. Poole CA, Ayad S, Gilbert RT (1992) Chondrons from articular cartilage – V. Immunohisto-chemical evaluation of type VI collagen organisation in isolated chondrons by light, confocal and electron microscopy. J Cell Sci 103:1101–1110

14. Schenk RK, Eggli PS, Hunziker EB (1986) Articular cartilage morphology. In: Kuettner K, Schleyerbach R, Hascall V (eds) Articular cartilage biochemistry. Raven Press, New York, pp3–22

15. Söder S, Hambach L, Lissner R, Kirchner T, Aigner T (2002) Ultrastructural localization of type VI collagen in normal adult and osteoarthritic human articular cartilage. Osteoarthritis Cartilage 10:464–470

CHAPTER 2

Cartilage Injury and Repair **2**

CHRISTIAN HENDRICH, NORBERT SCHÜTZE, THOMAS BARTHEL,
ULRICH NÖTH and JOCHEN EULERT

Cartilage Biology

Hyaline articular cartilage is composed of water (75%), matrix (20%), and cells (5%). The cells within the matrix are termed chondrocytes. The matrix consists of 80% collagen, with collagen type II being the major component accounting for approximately 90% of the total collagen content. Collagen type II is thought to be essential for the tensile stability of articular cartilage. The network formed by collagen type II is cross-linked by collagen type IX. Responsible for the high water-binding capacity and thus for the elastic properties of hyaline cartilage are proteoglycans, which form approximately 20% of the matrix [21]. The task of the chondrocytes is to secrete and maintain their surrounding matrix. Despite their relatively small volume the chondrocytes are the essential players in cartilage damage and repair. The specific organization with a small number of cells embedded in a large amount of matrix makes chondrocytes relatively inert against hypoxia. Because of the missing blood supply a significant inflammatory reaction does not occur after cartilage injury. Also, if a cartilage defect is not penetrating the subchondral bone the access to a reservoir of mesenchymal progenitor cells is not given and the chances for repair are limited [23].

Partial and Full-Thickness Defects

Cartilage lesions are classified as partial defects (without penetration of the subchondral bone) or full-thickness defects (with penetration of the subchondral bone). Partial defects have been examined using different animal models. In rabbits, a superficial laceration of the articular cartilage has shown neither healing nor progression over a 2-year time period [10]. However, in a similar model a more progressive degeneration has been observed [13]. Beside the limited regeneration on the cellular level it is thought that the negatively charged proteoglycans expressed on the injured cartilage surface hinder cellular adhesion. Interestingly, treatment of partial defects with chondroitinase ABC or trypsin solution resulted in a markedly enhanced repair by synovial cells in the rabbit and the mini pig [17, 18]. For the surgical treatment of partial defects it has to be considered that any kind of shaving of a superficial lesion is supposed to provoke further cartilage degeneration [24].

In full-thickness defects a fibrin clot forms within the defect after penetration of the subchondral bone. Cells from blood and bone marrow are bound within this clot and start to form islands of primitive cartilage. After approximately 6 to 12 weeks a layer of fibrous cartilage covers the defect surface. Initially, the matrix consists of collagen type I, which later gets partially replaced by collagen type II indicating a more hyaline-like tissue [8]. After one year, as known from studies in the rabbit the repair tissue shows the histological appearance of fibrocartilage including a tendency to superficial fibrillation [23, 26, 43]. In most animals a defect of 3 mm is thought to be of critical size meaning that no spontaneous healing can be expected [24]. Moreover, the healing capacity of a full-thickness defect is highly dependent on the age of the animal [40]. Although, many animal studies have served as useful tools studying articular cartilage repair mechanisms the natural course of cartilage healing in human remains unclear.

Debridement and Abrasion Arthroplasty

A simple arthroscopic lavage is known to give in only a temporal relief of the symptoms [6, 16]. Another technique is the arthroscopic debridement without penetrating the subchondral bone. In a study by Rand, the outcome of a debridement in 131 patients having grade III and IV cartilage lesions was compared to 34 patients having grade IV lesions and abrasion arthroplasty, with better results after debridement [37]. Bert and Maschka compared 67 patients (mean age 61 years) having a debridement to 59 patients (mean age 66 years) having an abrasion and also found better results after debridement [3]. However, the influence of the age difference was not discussed. A recent prospective and randomized study in a population of 165 veterans with a mean age of 52 years did not find a significant difference over a period of 24 months in patients having a lavage, a debridement, or a sham-operation [27] A controversial discussion whether the results of this study can be used in general has started.

Drilling and Microfracturing

A different approach is the penetration of the subchondral bone to induce a fibrous repair by mesenchymal progenitor cells from the bone marrow. Different techniques have been described. The original drilling technique described by Pridie and the complete removal of the subchondral plate as described by Ficat are resulting in a failure of the regenerate because of the weakening of the bony structure [6, 30]. Steadmans' microfracturing technique using special awls showed in 233 patients with an average age of 38 years and having grade IV cartilage lesions an improvement of pain in 75% and in activities of daily life in 65%. While over 7 years the results slowly deteriorated in only 9% of the patients a re-intervention was necessary. However, the results are not as good as in patients older than 30 years [42]. The possibility of an arthroscopic application at a low additional risk makes microfracturing a no-harm procedure [29]. A definitive statement about its efficiency and a comparison to osteochondral or chondrocyte transplantation is still missing [14] (see chapter 6).

Osteochondral Grafts and Autologous Chondrocyte Transplantation

The transplantation of osteochondral grafts and autologous chondrocytes is reviewed in individual chapters (see chapter 3 and 7). For osteochondral transplantation different techniques and instruments have been described. Long-term results are still missing. Hangody has found good to excellent results in 84 to 95% of the patients depending on the localization of the defect. However, a follow-up time is not reported. The upper age limit is considered at 50 years. The results in patients older than 35 years are less satisfactory [14]. The maximum size of the defect, the integration of the osteochondral cylinders, and the donor site morbidity are still under discussion.

The autologous chondrocyte transplantation (ACT) has been the first cell-based articular cartilage repair procedure described. Meanwhile excellent long-term results have been reported by Peterson et al. [31]. The upper age limit has been set to 55 years [15]. Biopsies taken from patients after ACT have shown excellent cartilage repair [38]. However, these clinical results could not be reproduced in an animal model [5]. The ACT has major impact on future orthopaedic tissue engineering concepts of articular cartilage repair.

Cartilage Tissue Engineering

Tissue engineering is the interdisciplinary application of principles from engineering and cell biology to generate tissues for restoration, maintenance, or replacement of lost organ functions. Tissue engineering concepts include the use of cells, matrices, and growth factors. In the ACT procedure different membranes made of collagen type I, a combination of collagen type I and III, and hyaluronic acid are commercially available as substitutes for the periostal flap [34] (see chapter 6 and 18). Also, chondrocytes are cultured on the membranes and fixed into the defect by fibrin glue. A number of these modified techniques just entered clinical trials. The future will show which technique is most beneficial for the patient.

Of major interest is the question whether chondrocytes can be replaced by multipotent mesenchymal stem cells (MSCs) [7]. MSCs can be isolated from many mesenchymal tissues, such as periosteum, adipose, muscle, trabecular bone, and bone marrow [32] (see chapter 15). Depending on the cell culture conditions MSCs can be differentiated into bone, muscle, fat or other tissues of mesenchymal origin. In the presence of growth factors, such as TGF-β the differentiation into cells of the chondrogenic lineage has been described [19, 44]. However, implantation of a tissue engineered device into humans after *in vitro* application of growth factors might require regulatory approval. While chondrocytes and MSCs have shown their chondrogenic differentiation potential a comparison of both cell types under *in vivo* conditions has not been performed yet (see chapter 20).

Cartilage Injury and Osteoarthritis

The process leading from an isolated cartilage lesion to an osteoarthritic lesion is not understood. A simple mechanical theory is the development of osteoarthritis as a result of mechanical wear by the ongoing use of the joint. In the normal joint cyclic loading leads to an enhanced synthesis of aggrecans. In contrast, the absence of motion and prolonged static loading is known to cause matrix degradation [6]. Also, a higher prevalence of osteoarthritis was found in patients working as constructors, farmers, and metal workers. High impact sports and activities with excessive shear forces are also believed to promote osteoarthritis [25]. In animal models repetitive direct impact and shear forces have shown morphological and biochemical signs of cartilage degradation [35, 36].

In the late stage of osteoarthritis all tissues of the joint are included in the pathologic process. In early osteoarthritis the primary events are the loss of cartilage, remodeling of the subchondral bone, and the formation of osteophytes. The process of cartilage loss is divided in three overlapping steps: the disruption of the matrix, the concomitant loss of chondrocytes with initially increased and later decreased synthetic activity, and the resulting progressive loss of cartilage tissue [6]. The main actor in this pathologic process is the chondrocyte. The degeneration process varies between individuals and among different joints. In most cases the progression is slow and goes over many years. The individual susceptibility is governed by numerous systemic and local biomechanical factors. The latter is often relevant for secondary osteoarthritis, such as observed in patients with obesity, joint injury, joint dysplasia or instability, sports activities, and conditions of muscle weakness [9, 20]. Also aging, as well as genetic and hormonal factors largely influence the onset and progression of the disease.

Cellular and Molecular Aspects

Local mediators and signal transduction pathways acting in the context of systemic factors contribute to the imbalance in synthesis and destruction of articular cartilage [33]. Enhanced catabolism of the articular cartilage in osteoarthritis is mediated by degradative proteases secreted from the chondrocyte [2]. Matrix metalloproteinases responsible for matrix turnover are activated by several mechanisms and regulated by cytokines, hormones, tissue inhibitors, and mechanical forces. Members include collagenases (MMP-1), gelatinases (MMP-2), stromelysin (MMP-3) and others, such as the ADAMTS-family (a disintegrin and metalloproteinase with thrombospondin motif). As a consequence of the proteolytic activities matrix breakdown products are released into the synovial fluid leading to the activation of synovial macrophages, which in turn results in the release of factors such as IL-1, TNFα, NO-radicals, and others. These local factors act on chondrocytes and alter their gene expression pattern resulting in changes of the anabolic and catabolic pathways. These mechanisms alter the activities of growth factors (IGF and TGF-ß etc.) and modulate the response of chondrocytes to cytokines and apoptosis [11, 12, 39]. Gene expression profiling studies have significantly contributed to the elucidation of novel pathways associated with osteoarthritis [1, 2]. Powerful molecular biology methods including genomics and proteomics will further enhance our knowledge of normal cartilage cell biology and alterations occurring in osteoarthritis in the near future.

Genetics and Osteoarthritis

Although research of the past years has led to a better understanding of the molecular events associated with the progression of osteoarthritis we are still far from a complete picture, particularly with regard to the mechanisms initiating the disease. From epidemiological studies, ethnic differences in the prevalence of primary osteoarthritis suggest a genetic component of the disease. This is supported by several genome studies [4]. Genetic factors contribute at least to 50% of the cases of osteoarthritis in hands and hips [41]. Linkage analysis identified a number of genome regions although LOD-scores often have been relatively low [4, 22, 28]. Some regions have been linked to osteoarthritis by several independent studies, such as regions on the chromosomes 2q and 11q and therefore could have a significant relevance. It is likely that different chromosomal regions harbor genes which are important for subgroups of osteoarthritis. In the future, additional chromosomal areas will be identified and genes within identified regions will be characterized, which should enhance our understanding of the initiation and progression of the disease.

In theory, all genes which encode proteins with significant function in the different cells types of the joint can be seen as candidate genes. Functional polymorphisms within these gene regions could contribute to the individual susceptibility to osteoarthritis. Although the results of association studies of polymorphisms have been discussed controversial in the past [4]. With improvements such as higher numbers of patients and more careful selection of patients we can expect the identification of additional disease-associated functional polymorphisms. Further functional genomic studies and gene expression profiling analysis should lead to a better understanding of osteoarthritis.

Summary

Different articular cartilage repair techniques for chondral and full-thickness defects are currently in clinical use or at an experimental stage of development. Most promising future technologies are coming from the relatively new field of tissue engineering, especially the use of cell-based articular cartilage repair strategies. The mechanisms leading to the osteoarthitic cartilage lesion are multifactorial. Further functional genomic studies and gene expression profiling analysis should identify new targets for therapeutic interventions and should provide perspectives for an individual risk analysis.

References

1. Aigner T, Bartnik E, Zien A, Zimmer R (2002) Functional genomics of osteoarthritis. Pharmacogenomics 3:635–650
2. Aigner T, Kurz B, Fukui N, Sandell L (2002) Roles of chondrocytes in the pathogenesis of osteoarthritis. Curr Opin Rheumatol 14:578–584
3. Bert JM, Maschka K (1989) The arthroscopic treatment of unicompartimental gonarthrosis: a five-year follow-up study of abrasion arthroplasty plus arthroscopic debridement and arthroscopic debridement alone. Arthroscopy 5:25–32

4. Brandi ML, Gennari L, Cerinic MM et al. (2001) Genetic markers of osteoarticular disorders: facts and hopes. Arthritis Res 3:270–280

5. Breinan HA, Minas T, Hsu HP, Nehrer S, Sledge CB, Spector M (1997) Effect of cultured autologous chondrocytes on repair of chondral defects in a canine model. J Bone Joint Surg-A 79:1439–1451

6. Buckwalter JA, Mankin HJ (1998) Articular cartilage: degeneration and osteoarthritis, repair, regeneration, and transplantation. Instr Course Lect 47:487–504

7. Caplan AI, Elyaderani M, Mochizuki Y, Wakitani S, Goldberg VM (1997) Principles of cartilage repair and regeneration. Clin Orthop 342:254–269

8. Cheung HS, Cottrell WH, Stephenson K, Nimni ME (1978) In vitro collagen biosynthesis in healing and normal rabbit articular cartilage. J Bone Joint Surg-A 60:1076–1081

9. Felson DT, Lawrence RC, Hochberg MC et al. (2000) Osteoarthritis: new insights. Part 1: the disease and its risk factors. Ann Intern Med 133:635–646

10. Ghadially FN, Thomas I, Oryschak AF, Lalonde JM (1977) Long-term results of superficial defects in articular cartilage: a scanning electron-microscope study. J Pathol 121:213–217

11. Ghosh P, Smith M (2002) Osteoarthritis, genetic and molecular mechanisms. Biogerontology 3:85–88

12. Goldring MB (2000) Osteoarthritis and cartilage: the role of cytokines. Curr Rheumatol Rep 2:459–465

13. Grande DA, Pitman MI, Peterson L, Menche D, Klein M (1989) The repair of experimentally produced defects in rabbit articular cartilage by autologous chondrocyte transplantation. J Orthop Res 7:208–218

14. Hangody L (2001) Mosaicplasty. In: Insall JN, Scott WN (eds) Surgery of the knee, vol 1, 3rd edn. Churchill Livingstone, Philadelphia, pp357–350

15. Hjelle K, Solheim E, Strand T, Muri R, Brittberg M et al. (2002) Articular cartilage defects in 1,000 knee arthroscopies. Arthroscopy 18:730–734

16. Hubbard MJ (1987) Arthroscopic surgery for chondral flaps in the knee. J Bone Joint Surg-Br 69:794–796

17. Hunziker EB, Kapfinger E (1998) Removal of proteoglycans from the surface of defects in articular cartilage transiently enhances coverage by repair cells. J Bone Joint Surg-Br 80:144–150

18. Hunziker EB, Rosenberg LC (1996) Repair of partial-thickness defects in articular cartilage: cell recruitment from the synovial membrane. J Bone Joint Surg-A 78:721–733

19. Johnstone B, Hering TM, Caplan AI, Goldberg VM, Yoo JU (1998) In vitro chondrogenesis of bone marrow-derived mesenchymal progenitor cells. Exp Cell Res 238:265–272

20. Kerin A, Patwari P, Kuettner K, Cole A, Grodzinsky A (2002) Molecular basis of osteoarthritis: biomechanical aspects. Cell Mol Life Sci 59:27–35

21. Kuettner KE (1992) Biochemistry of articular cartilage in health and disease. Clin Biochem 25:155–163

22. Loughlin J (2001) Genetic epidemiology of primary osteoarthritis. Curr Opin Rheumatol 13:111–116

23. Mankin HJ (1982) The response of articular cartilage to mechanical injury. J Bone Joint Surg-A 64:460–466

24. Messner K (2001) Healing of articular cartilage injuries. In: Insall JN, Scott WN (eds) Surgery of the knee, vol 1, 3rd edn. Churchill Livingstone, Philadelphia, pp327–340

25. Messner K, Maletius W (1996) The long-term prognosis for severe damage to weight-bearing cartilage in the knee: a 14-year clinical and radiographic follow-up in 28 young athletes. Acta Orthop Scand 67:165–168

26. Mitchell N, Shepard N (1976) The resurfacing of adult rabbit articular cartilage by multiple perforations through the subchondral bone. J Bone Joint Surg-A 58:230–233

27. Moseley JB, O'Malley K, Peterson NJ et al. (2002) A controlled trial of arthroscopic surgery for osteoarthritis of the knee. N Engl J Med 347:81–88

28. Newman B, Wallis GA (2002) Is osteoarthritis a genetic disease? Clin Invest Med 25:139–149

29. O'Driscoll SW (1998) The healing and regeneration of articular cartilage. J Bone Joint Surg-A 80:1795–1812

30. Peterson L (2001) International experience with autologous chondrocyte transplantation. In: Insall JN, Scott WN (eds) Surgery of the knee, vol 1, 3rd edn. Churchill Livingstone, Philadelphia, pp341–356
31. Peterson L, Minas T, Brittberg M, Nilsson A, Sjogren-Jansson E, Lindahl A (2000) Two- to 9-year outcome after autologous chondrocyte transplantation of the knee. Clin Orthop 374:212–234
32. Pittenger MF, Mackay AM, Beck SC et al. (1999) Multilineage potential of adult human mesenchymal stem cells. Science 284:143–147
33. Pullig O, Pfander D, Swoboda B (2001) Molecular principles of induction and progression of arthrosis. Orthopäde 30:825–833
34. Radice M, Brun P, Cortivo R, Scapinelli R, Battaliard C, Abatangelo G (2000) Hyaluronan-based biopolymers as delivery vehicles for bonemarrow-derived mesenchymal progenitors. J Biomed Mater Res 50:101–109
35. Radin EL, Ehrlich MG, Chernack R, Abernethy P, Paul IL, Rose RM (1978) Effect of repetitive impulsive loading on the knee joints of rabbits. Clin Orthop 131:288–293
36. Radin EL, Martin RB, Burr DB, Caterson B, Boyd RD, Goodwin C (1984) Effects of mechanical loading on the tissues of the rabbit knee. J Orthop Res 2:221–234
37. Rand JA (1991) Role of arthroscopy in osteoarthritis of the knee. Arthroscopy 7:358–363
38. Roberts S, Hollander AP, Caterson B, Menage J, Richardson JB (2001) Matrix turnover in human cartilage repair tissue in autologous chondrocyte implantation. Arthritis Rheum 44:2586–2598
39. Sharma L (2001) Local factors in osteoarthritis. Curr Opin Rheumatol 13:441–446
40. Solchaga LA, Goldberg VM, Caplan AI (2001) Cartilage regeneration using principles of tissue engineering. Clin Orthop 391 [Suppl]:S161–S170
41. Spector TD, Cicuttini F, Baker J, Loughlin J, Hart D (1996) Genetic influences on osteoarthritis in women: a twin study. BMJ 312:940–943
42. Steadman JR et al. (2001) Debridement and microfracture ("Pick Technique") for full-thickness articular cartilage defects. In: Insall JN, Scott WN (eds) Surgery of the knee, vol 1, 3rd edn. Churchill Livingstone, Philadelphia, pp361–373
43. Wei X, Gao J, Messner K (1997) Maturation-dependent repair of untreated osteochondral defects in the rabbit knee joint. J Biomed Mater Res 34:63–72
44. Yoo JU, Barthel DS, Nishimura K, Solchaga L, Caplan AI, Goldberg VM, Johnstone B (1998) The chondrogenic potential of human bonemarrow-derived mesenchymal progenitor cells. J Bone Joint Surg-A 80:1745–1757

Clinical Results

II

CHAPTER 3

Autologous Chondrocyte Transplantation (ACT) – Long-Term Results

3

LARS PETERSON

Problems associated with the treatment of an injury to the hyaline articular cartilage are known since a long time and are still greatly discussed [6]. An injury that extends through all layers of cartilage down to the subchondral bone, or even through the bone, is likely to progress to osteoarthritis by degradation through a combination of mechanical wear and enzymatic digestion [3]. To detect and treat a cartilage injury at an early stage before it leads to a vast joint destruction is therefore of outmost importance. Current therapies including drilling, abrasion and microfracturing are introducing mesenchymal progenitor cells from the bone marrow to provide a repair tissue. However, this repair tissue may end up in fibrous tissue, which over time will not stand wear and load of the joint. Buckwalter stated in 1990 "the ultimate measure of cartilage repair must be the degree of restoration of synovial joint function following an injury that alters joint function meaning not necessarily repair tissue of identical morphological structure" [4].

It seems however to be important to define and differ between tissue repair and regeneration. Repair of cartilage means replacing the damaged tissue with new but not identical tissue. Regeneration of cartilage means replacing the damaged tissue with new tissue identical to the original. It seems optimal to provide a tissue not only restoring the synovial joint function but also a tissue that stands the wear and tear over time. Regeneration of tissue integrated in the normal turnover of cartilage seems more likely to fulfill these criteria and should be the aim of our treatment.

The present use of MSC-based techniques shows good short-term results but we still lack long-term results and objective evaluation of the resulting repair tissue. Autologous chondrocyte transplantation (ACT) is using articular chondrocytes isolated and grown in culture in the first attempt to heal a cartilage lesion with hyaline cartilage, to regenerate cartilage. The articular chondrocyte is the only cell committed to produce hyaline cartilage. ACT has been elaborated in extensive animal work since 1982 [2, 5, 12] and used clinically since 1987, with the approval of the Ethical Committee of the Medical Faculty of the University of Gothenburg. Over 1200 patients have been operated in Gothenburg and over an additional 8000 worldwide since 1995.

Autologous chondrocyte transplantation (ACT) is a two-stage procedure and is indicated for treating symptomatic full-thickness cartilage lesions covering an area of 1 to 16 cm^2 on the femur and the patella. The treatment has mainly been used in the knee but has also been tried in the ankle, the hip, the shoulder, and the MCP joint of the thumb; henceforth the article refers to the knee joint.

The patients have been evaluated with subjective and objective ratings: Lysholm score, patient and physician modified Cincinnati rating system, Brittberg-Peterson functional assessment score and Wallgren-Tegner activity score, as well as an overall clinical rating and arthroscopic assessment of the repair tissue. Indentation tests of the stiffness of the repair tissue, evaluation of histological appearance and immunohistochemical analysis of biopsies from the repair tissue were performed. In this chapter I will focus on the long-term results of a cohort of 61 patients.

Surgical Techniques

Chondral Lesions

The first step of the procedure is an arthroscopic assessment of the joint including the synovial lining, the menisci, the cruciate ligaments, and all articulating surfaces. The articular lesion including the bony defect (osteochondritis dissecans; OCD) is evaluated and documented regarding location, size, depth, containment, and quality of the surrounding cartilage. The opposing cartilage surface should have no or only minor damage. The International Cartilage Repair Society (ICRS) has designed forms for documentation of the cartilage lesions. If ACT is assessed appropriate for the lesion small specimens of cartilage are harvested from the proximal medial edge of the trochlea. The specimens are sent to the laboratory for cell isolation and culture of the chondrocytes in a medium including the patient's own serum for two weeks [1].

The second step includes an arthrotomy or mini-arthrotomy whenever possible. Depending on the location of the lesion a medial or lateral arthrotomy is used. The arthrotomy is adjusted so the lesion is adequately accessed. A knife is used to incise around all damaged and fissured cartilage, which is then debrided. The debridement has to be done very carefully and all damaged cartilage has to be removed without causing any bleeding to the subchondral bone. A bleeding may result in migration of undifferentiated progenitor cells from the bone marrow that may form a repair tissue of fibrous character.

When all pathologic cartilage is removed and vertical edges to stable healthy cartilage are present the lesion should be covered with a periosteal flap. For correct form and size of the flap a template of the cartilage lesion is made. Periosteum is exposed at a separate incision at the proximal medial tibia and is carefully dissected free from fat and fibrous tissue. The template is used when incising for accurate size of the periosteal flap by adding 1 to 2 mm at the periphery. It is important that the cambium layer is included and still attached to the periosteum, so the flap has to be detached very carefully. The flap is placed on top of the lesion with the cambium layer facing the defect and interrupted resorbable 6.0 sutures are used at 3 to 5 mm intervals to secure the flap to the cartilage edge and thus tensioning it like the skin of a drum over the defect. However, a superior opening is left for injecting the chondrocytes. The intervals between the sutures are sealed with fibrin glue. Saline is gently injected underneath the periosteal flap to check for leakage between the flap and the cartilage rim. If no leakage can be detected the saline is aspirated and the chondrocytes in suspension are injected to fill the defect completely. The last opening is closed and the wound is sutured in layers [7, 9, 10] (Fig. 3.1).

Osteochondral Lesions

When treating a shallow osteochondral lesion with a bony defect no deeper than 6 to 8 mm the sclerotic bottom of the bony defect is debrided, again very carefully so no bleeding is caused. Then the procedure follows that for chondral lesions (Fig. 3.2).

However, if the bony defect is deeper additional steps have to be taken to restore the contour of the bone. The sclerotic bottom of the defect is abraded and multiple drilling down to the bone marrow is performed. The bony defect is filled with cancellous bone and then covered with a periosteal flap at the level of the subchondral bone with the cambium layer facing the joint. You then go forth with the transplantation of the chondrocytes as if treating a chondral lesion [8] (Fig. 3.3).

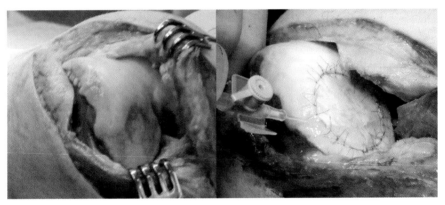

Fig. 3.1. Chondral lesion (*left*) that is treated with ACT (*right*).

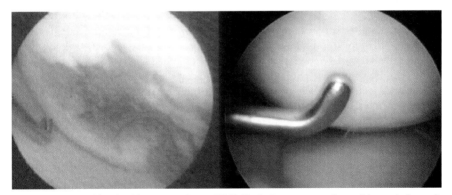

Fig. 3.2. 17-year old girl with OCD. Before ACT (*left*). Arthroscopy performed by an independent orthopaedic surgeon one year after treatment with ACT (*right*). Excellent clinical result 6 years after treatment.

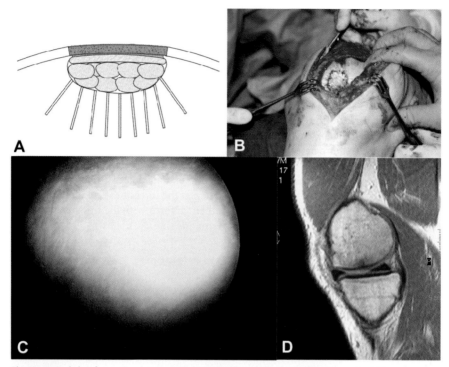

Fig. 3.3A–D. (A) Schematic picture with bone graft (*gray*), fibrin glue (*green*) and between two periosteal flaps (*red*) chondrocytes in suspension (*blue*). **(B)** Treatment of a deep OCD with concomitant autologous bone graft and chondrocyte transplantation. **(C)** Second-look arthroscopy reveals filling with repair tissue. **(D)** MRI at 38 months after treatment shows reestablishment of the bony contour covered with cartilage.

Rehabilitation

Six to 8 hours after surgery the patient starts passive motion training using a CPM-machine with 0° to 30° (or 40°) of motion. Quadriceps and active ROM-training starts the day after surgery. The weight-bearing on the operated leg has to be partial for the first weeks. How much weight is allowed depends on the size, location, and number of transplanted defects and concomitant procedures. The weight-bearing ranges from weight-bearing to the pain threshold for the first 6 weeks for a small contained lesion on the femoral condyle, to 30 to 40 pounds for 6 to 8 weeks, then gradually increasing the weight-bearing up to full weight-bearing within the following 6 weeks for large lesions or multiple lesions with concomitant procedures.

Training on a stationary bike can be performed when the wound is healed and the needed knee flexion is achieved, a low resistance is used. Encourage bicycling during the whole rehabilitation program. When the wound is healed you can start training in water. When full weight-bearing is achieved increased walking distances are encouraged. If possible use skating, inline skating or cross-country skiing on even surfaces as an intermediate training before returning to running. Running should be postponed 6 to 9 months and started on an individual basis.

Return to professional athletic training and competition should be judged on an individual basis including assessment of ROM, muscle strength and endurance, arthroscopic evaluation, and probing of the repaired area.

Earlier Results

The results of the first 23 patients were presented in the New England Journal of Medicine in 1994 [1]. These results were encouraging for patients with defects of the femoral condyle, but from the 7 patients with patellar lesions only 2 were considered good or excellent. Today the technique has been improved not only in femoral condyle lesions but also in patellar lesions and OCD of the femoral condyle that extends down through the subchondral bone. This has been achieved by considering factors such as ligament instability, patellar malalignment, deep bony defects, varus or valgus deformity, and meniscus deficiency in addition to the chondral lesion.

In Gothenburg, 219 patients were followed for 2 to 9 years after surgery [13]. This study included the patients from the first study and patients operated thereafter, in total 213 were assessed. Attention was paid and action was taken to correct background factors as mentioned. When evaluating the patients they where divided into five groups: isolated cartilage lesion on the medial or lateral femoral condyle (isolated FC), multiple cartilage lesions (multiple lesions), OCD on the femoral condyle (OCD), patella lesion that also needed surgical realignment of the patella (patella), and femoral condyle lesion with concomitant anterior cruciate ligament reconstruction (FC + ACL). The group that responded best to the ACT procedure was the isolated FC lesions with 92% of the patients showing improvement at a 2 to 9 year follow-up. In the OCD group 89% of the patients considered themselves improved by the surgical procedure and in the patellar group 68%. Surprisingly, the multiple lesion group graded well with 67% showing improvement. In the multiple lesion patient the surgery is often performed as a salvage procedure since the patient is relatively young with grave damage to the knee joint and thus the treatment options are very limited (Fig 3.4).

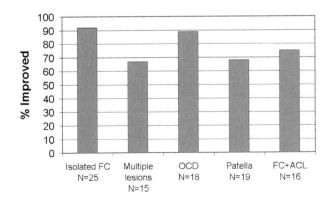

Fig. 3.4.
Improvement over 2 to 9 years after ACT.

Long-Term Results and Durability

Recently a long-term follow-up was published [11]. The status 2 years post ACT of the first 61 patients was compared to follow-ups of the same patients between 5 and 11 years (mean 7.4). The patient groups studied were isolated femoral condyle lesion, OCD on the femoral condyle, patellar lesion, and femoral condyle lesion with ACL reconstruction. The patients were clinically graded as poor, fair, good, or excellent [1]. The isolated femoral condyle group showed 89% good or excellent results after the 2-year follow-up and similar results at the 7.4-year follow-up. OCD lesions showed equally 86% good or excellent results at the 2 and 7.4 year follow-up. The patella group had increased in numbers from 7 to 17 and the good or excellent results went from 28% in 1994 to 65% in 2000 and to 76% in 2002. This study shows that if ACT gives a good or excellent result at a 2-year follow-up the results are durable 5 to 11 years after surgery (Fig. 3.5).

Recently, at the ICRS meeting in Toronto in 2002 results 3 to 13 years (mean 3.9) after ACT including more unusual injury locations of the knee were presented. Patients with lesions of the femoral trochlea were clinically assessed and 80% were considered good or excellent (Fig. 3.6). The group with multiple lesions of different compartments

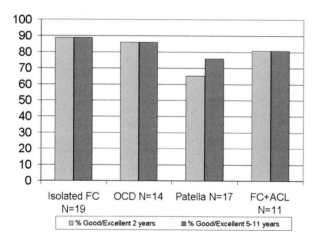

Fig. 3.5.
Clinical results 2 and 5 to 11 years after ACT.

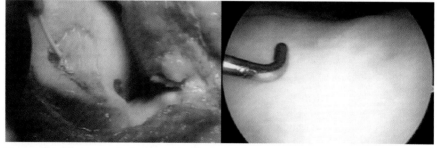

Fig. 3.6. Trochlea groove lesion treated with ACT (*left*). Arthroscopy performed 2.5 years after surgery showing a complete filling of the defect (*right*). Excellent clinical result.

of the knee showed 84% good or excellent results. Multiple lesions of the same compartment on the femur and tibia showed 75% good or excellent results (Fig. 3.6).

Assessments

Arthroscopic Assessment

Second-look arthroscopy was done in 46 patients and a macroscopic assessment of the repair tissue according to the degree of defect filling (0 to 4 points), integration to border zone (0 to 4 points), and macroscopic appearance (0 to 4 points) was performed. Optimal results of 12 points equaled perfect filling, integration and surface appearance. The results were for isolated femoral condyle lesions 10.3, isolated femoral condyle with ACL reconstruction 10.9, and OCD 10.5.

Histological Assessment

Biopsies analyzed by independent pathologists showed hyaline-like cartilage in 80% of the samples (Fig. 3.6).

Immunohistochemical Assessment

Immunohistochemical analysis of 29 biopsies showed ++ to +++ for collagen type II, COMP, and aggrecan compared to +++ for normal cartilage (Table 3.1).

Biomechanical Indentation Assessment

Indentation tests of normal cartilage and repair tissue using an electromechanical indentation probe (Artscan Inc, Kuopio, Finland) was performed arthroscopically by

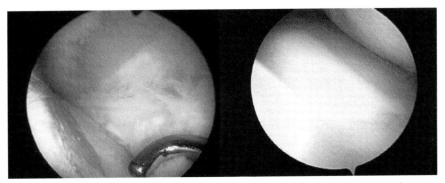

Fig. 3.7. 39-year old woman with bipolar medial compartment bone to bone lesions before ACT (*left*) and arthroscopy 15 months after ACT (*right*).

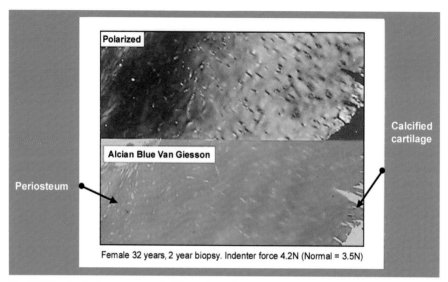

Fig. 3.8. Histological assessment of a biopsy from the repair tissue showing hyaline cartilage-like characteristics.

Table 3.1. Immunohistochemical evaluation of 22 biopsies performed by independent pathologists

	Normal hyaline cartilage	Repair: fibrous cartilage	Repair: hyaline cartilage
Type I	$- \rightarrow (+)$	$++ \rightarrow +++$	$- \rightarrow (+)$
Type II	$+++$	$-$	$++ \rightarrow +++$
COMP	$+++$	$+ \rightarrow ++$	$++ \rightarrow +++$
Aggrecan	$+++$	$+ \rightarrow ++$	$++ \rightarrow +++$
n =	3	6	13

an unbiased examiner. The stiffness was measured in normal cartilage and the repaired area. Biopsies were taken from the center of the repaired area. There was no significant difference between normal cartilage stiffness and that of the repaired tissue (Fig. 3.9).

Conclusion

ACT has been in clinical use for over 15 years. The overall good to excellent results are 84% at 2 years follow-up and remain good to excellent at 5 to 11 years follow-up with excellent durability. Even patellofemoral lesions can get acceptable results when background factors are corrected. The subjective results are supported by independent clinicians evaluation along with macroscopic, microscopic, immunohistochemical and biomechanical assessments.

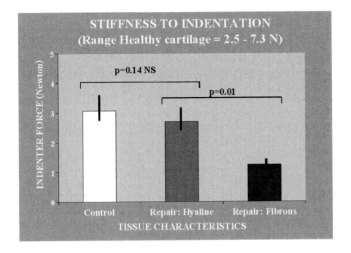

Fig. 3.9.
Biomechanical indentation assessment.

References

1. Brittberg M, Lindahl A, Nilsson A et al. (1994) Treatment of deep cartilage defects in the knee with autologous chondrocyte transplantation. N Engl J Med 331:889–895
2. Brittberg M, Nilsson M, Lindahl A et al. (1996) Rabbit articular cartilage defects treated with autologous cultured chondrocytes. Clin Orthop 326:270–283
3. Buckwalter JA, Mankin HJ (1997) Articular cartilage: Degeneration and osteoarthrosis, repair, regeneration and transplantation. J Bone Joint Surg-A 79:612–632
4. Buckwalter JA, Rosenberg LC, Hunziker EB (1990) Articular cartilage: Composition, structure, response to injury and methods of facilitating repair. In: Ewing JW (ed) Articular cartilage and knee joint function: basic science and arthroscopy. Raven Press, New York, pp19–56
5. Grande DA, Pitman MI, Peterson L et al. (1989) The repair of experimentally produced defects in rabbit articular cartilage by autologous chondrocyte transplantation. J Orthop Res 7:208–218
6. Hunter W (1743) On the structure and disease of articular cartilage. Philos Trans R Soc Lond 42d:514–521
7. Minas T, Peterson L (1999) Advanced techniques in autologous chondrocyte transplantation. Clin Sports Med 18:13–44
8. Peterson L (2002) Technique of autologous chondrocyte transplantation. Tech Knee Surg 1:2–12
9. Peterson L (2001) International experience with autologous chondrocyte transplantation. In: Insall JN, Scott WN (eds) Surgery of the knee, vol 1, 3rd edn. Churchill Livingstone, Philadelphia, pp341–356
10. Peterson L (2001) Cartilage cell transplantation. In: Malek (ed) Knee surgery, complications, pitfalls and salvage. Springer, New York, pp440–449
11. Peterson L, Brittberg M, Kiwiranta I, et al (2002) Autologous chondrocyte transplantation: Biomechanics and long-term durability. Am J Sports Med 30:2–12
12. Peterson L, Menche D, Grande D et al. (1984) Chondrocyte transplantation: an experimental model in the rabbit. Trans Orthop Res Soc 30:218
13. Peterson L, Minas T, Brittberg M et al. (2000) Two- to 9-year outcome after autologous chondrocyte transplantation of the knee. Clin Orthop 374:212–234

EURACT Study: A 24-Month Follow-up Multicenter Study of 84 Knees Treated with Autologous Chondrocyte Transplantation (ACT)

4

SVEN ANDERS, JENS SCHAUMBURGER, JOHANNES LÖHNERT
and JOACHIM GRIFKA*

Introduction

The unique mechanical and biochemical properties of hyaline articular cartilage reflect its high-end functional specification, which is provided by a complex histo-architecture [6, 7, 17, 26]. Therefore, structural cartilage integrity is inevitable for sufficient joint function. Low metabolism and an insufficient self-repair capacity make articular cartilage vulnerable for structural alteration. Any disarrangement of the articular homeostasis by single or repetitive exogenous and/or endogenous factors evokes cascade-like cellular and humoral interactions with little restitution but structural disarrangement [8, 9, 20]. Isolated lesions or degenerative loss of hyaline cartilage substance necessarily leads to joint degeneration and arthritis.

Autologous Chondrocyte Transplantation

Autologous chondrocyte transplantation (ACT) is a cell-based tissue engineering method for chondrocyte-induced cartilage repair. Except for the transplantation of osteochondral grafts (OCT) only ACT provides the capacity for articular cartilage repair resulting in hyaline or hyaline-like tissue [15]. In contrast to OCT, cell amplification *in vitro* and *de novo* chondrogenesis *in vivo* are key features of this technique. Animal trials using ACT were started in the early 80's [13]. The clinical application in human was published by Brittberg and Peterson in 1994 and today nearly 8000 ACT procedures have been performed [4, 5, 10, 25]. Preliminary results of the EURACT study using chondrotransplant® (co.don®-AG, Teltow, Germany) have been published [14, 18]. The results of a 24-month follow-up are presented here.

* Participants in the EURACT study: J. Beyer (Apollo-Klinik, Stuttgart, Germany), S. Feldt (co.don® AG, Teltow, Germany), H. Hornung (Martin-Luther-Krankenhaus, Berlin, Germany), G. Kleemann (Radiologische Praxis, Duisburg, Germany), H. Kniffler (Orthopädische Praxis, Kelkheim, Germany), S. Philippou (Augusta-Kranken-Anstalten Bochum, Germany), J. Scholz (Auguste-Viktoria-Krankenhaus, Berlin, Germany), M. Thomsen (Orthopädische Klinik AK Barmbek, Hamburg, Germany), H. Toutenburg (Institut für Statistik, Universität München, Germany).

Material and Methods

Patients

The prospective EURACT multicenter study reviews the outcome of 82 patients with 84 focal articular cartilage defects (partial or full-thickness) of the medial or lateral femoral condyle, the trochlea or the patella treated with the ACT procedure. Exclusion criteria were defects of the tibia plateau, opposing femoral and tibial lesions, generalized osteoarthritis, total meniscectomy, limb axis deformities, overweight, and patients older than 55 years. The cartilage biopsy was harvested arthroscopically and processed under standardized conditions. The cell culture procedure was performed according to the German drug law using the patient's own serum. No growth factors, antibiotics or antimycotics were added [12]. The transplantation of the cells was performed 2 to 4 weeks after biopsy using a mini-arthrotomy [14]. Clinical controls at 6 weeks, 3, 6, and 12 months after surgery were scheduled. MRI using cartilage adapted sequence parameters were performed after 6 and 12 months.

Clinical Scores

For evaluation the modified Cincinnati score [3], Lysholm score [19], HSS score [21], DGKKT score [18], and the Wallgren-Tegner activity score [28] were used. The results were transferred to a four point scale (1 = poor, 2 = far, 3 = good, and 4 = excellent). A ten point visual analogous scale (VAS; 0 = very unsatisfied, 10 = very satisfied) for the patients' self-assessment was implemented. The mean of all categorized scores (except Tegner) was transferred to a combined score which was standardized with four grades (1 = poor to 4 = excellent).

Second-Look Arthroscopy

In case of postoperative complaints or clinical symptoms like locking, swelling or edema a second-look arthroscopy was performed. The gross appearance of the repair tissue concerning its integration to the adjacent cartilage, the degree of defect filling, the surface structure and consistence was categorized into six groups: very good, very good/good, good, good/fair, fair, and fair/poor. In some cases a full-thickness needle biopsy was taken from the center of the repair tissue. This biopsy was examined histologically using HE and PAS staining. Immunohistochemical analysis for different collagen types to identify hyaline, hyaline-like or fibrocartilage was performed.

MRI

The degree of the defect filling, the signal difference of the repair tissue compared to the adjacent cartilage, the subchondral edema and joint effusion were rated with 0 to 2 points in each category with a maximum score of 12 points.

Statistical Analysis

The primary efficiency parameter was the healing rate within 24 months following ACT. Assessed as at least good by the modified Cincinnati score a patient was estimated as healed. The healing rates were analyzed for the other scores in an identical manner. In addition, a sum score was calculated as a combination of all scores except for the Wallgren-Tegner activity score to give a general evaluation of the patient's status at each time point. Finally, the correlation of the scores, the arthroscopical and radiological results, and the patient's age were analyzed using the Spearman's ranking correlation coefficient.

Study Population

The demographic data are shown in Table 4.1. No history of previous surgery was found in 50.6% of the cases. In pretreated patients (n = 39) an average of 2.3 surgical procedures (min = 1, max = 5) had been performed (15 patients without categorization): cartilage shaving (11 cases), bone-marrow stimulating techniques (e.g. drilling/microfracturing, 12 cases), partial meniscectomy (5 cases), OCT (3 cases), correction osteotomy (2 cases), ACL reconstruction (2 cases), and other procedures (4 cases). Poor results were seen in 52 patients (68.4%) and 21 patients (27.6%) had a moderate score result according to the modified Cincinnati score. The Wallgren-Tegner activity score was 1.9 ± 1.0 preoperatively (n = 78).

Results

Scores

The healing rate in the modified Cincinnati score was 61.4% after 12 months, 66.9% after 18 months and 82.2% after 24 months. The other scores exceeded these results at corresponding follow-ups (Fig. 4.1). The scores transferred to a four point scale showed a significant correlation for each category. The combined score reflected good (34/84

Table 4.1. Demographic Data

	Mean ± SD	Number of cases [n]
Age [years]	34.1 ± 9.7	84
Male/female	56/28	84
Defect size (cumulative for multiple lesions) [cm²]	4.5 ± 2.1	84
Medial/lateral condyle		51/13
Patella/trochlea		5/6
Multiple lesions		9
Chondral/osteochondral		51/33

= 41%) and very good (38/45 = 45%) results in 72/84 cases (86%), and fair (9/84 = 11%) or poor (3/84 = 3%) results in 12/84 (16%) cases. The Wallgren-Tegner activity score increased to 4.1 ± 0.9 after 24 months. The results of the sum score were not dependend on the defect localization (Fig. 4.2).

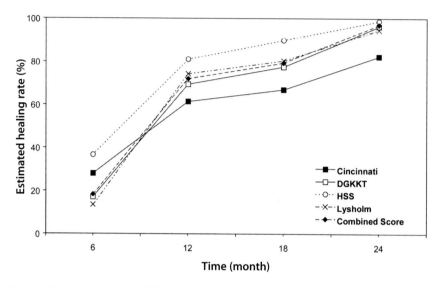

Fig. 4.1. Healing rates for the different scores and combined score (assessed by analysis of survival times using the method of Kaplan and Meier).

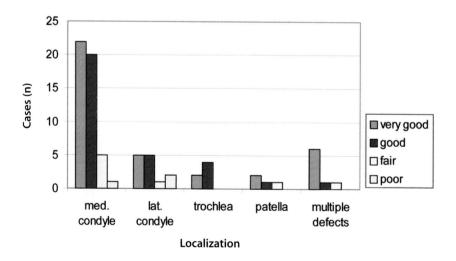

Fig. 4.2. Postoperative sum scores according to the defect localization.

MRI

In 66 cases a MRI at a mean time of 13.9 ± 6.4 months was performed postoperatively. The mean score was 5.8 points. In 60 cases (89.5%) had a good or excellent result with a score of at least 5 points.

Second-Look Arthroscopy

In 30 cases patients underwent a second-look arthroscopy at a mean of 11.4 ± 6.2 months after ACT. In 80% (24/30) the repair tissue formation was classified as good to very good, in 13.3% (4/30) as good/fair, and in 6.7% (2/30) as fair or fair/poor. The 14 optional biopsies were done 14.7 ± 6.4 months after ACT. They were categorized as hyaline or hyaline-like cartilage in 8 cases (57%), partial hyaline in 3 cases (21.4%), hyaline-fibrocartilage in 2 cases (14.2%), and as fibrocartilage in 1 case (7.1%). Six months after ACT a chondrocyte-like phenotype with a rare expression of collagen type I and distinct collagen type II expression was seen. Formation of chondron-like structures was seen after 15 months.

Patients Self-Evaluation

The mean satisfaction grade was 7.6 ± 2.5 points (n = 69) on the 10 point VAS. With a minimum of 6 points, 79.7% (55/69) of the patients were satisfied with the ACT procedure. The maximum of 10 points was given by 31.9% (22/69) patients. Sixty out of 68 patients (88.2%) recommended the ACT procedure, 8 patients (11.8%) did not. There was no correlation to gender or age.

Complications

Eleven from 84 cases (13%) had relevant complications and further treatment was necessary. Two had wound-healing problems and were treated conservatively. The other 9 cases had to undergo second-look arthroscopy and 2 partial periosteal delaminations, 1 regenerate tissue loosening and 1 regenerate tissue hypertrophy were identified as ACT-specific complications (5.9%). The other 4 cases had adhesions (2 cases), loose bodies (1 case), or trauma (1 case), and therefore were not classified as ACT-specific (4.7%).

Correlations

At the time of the ACT there was no significant correlation between the patients age and the modified Cincinnati score (p = 0.503) or the other scores. Whereas the health status at baseline was independent of the patient's age correlation between score and age was significant after 18 months (p <0.05). Older patients showed a prolonged rehabilitation. Chondral or osteochondral defects showed no statistical difference in these categories.

Summary

In this study, the treatment of focal cartilage defects of the knee joint with an average size of 4.5 cm^2 by ACT provided a healing rate of 61.4% after 12 months and 82.2% after 24 months, according to the modified Cincinnati score. The outcome in a combined four point scale showed 86% good (41%) or very good (45%) results. Arthroscopical, histological and MRI evaluation and patients self-assessment showed similar results. No statistical difference was found between the outcome of chondral and osteochondral defects. The patients self-assessment and histological classification of the repair tissue correlated significantly with the score results. The quality of the repair tissue seems to be essential for a normal joint function. The patients outcome was independent from the defect localization and depth. Neither the number nor the type of previous surgery did effect the results. The complication rate was comparable with those described in the literature [10, 11].

Conclusion

The periosteum-based ACT is a safe and efficient method for the repair of focal cartilage defects of the knee joint and results in an adequate hyaline or hyaline-like repair tissue. In nearly half of the cases it seems to be the method of first choice even after previous surgery. The authors recommend the ACT procedure for focal partial or full-thickness chondral or osteochondral defects with a size of more than 1 cm^2 with respect to the general accepted inclusion criteria [1]. The outcome of the ACT procedure with 70–96% of good or very good results and an up to 10 year follow-up was described by different authors [2, 10, 16, 18, 22–24, 27]. Nevertheless, well designed long-term studies are needed for further evaluation.

References

1. Anders S, Schaumburger J, Grifka J (2001) Surgical intra-articular interventions in arthrosis. Orthopäde 30:866–880
2. Bahuaud J, Maitrot RC, Bouvet R et al. (1998) Implantation of autologous chondrocytes for cartilagenous lesions in young patients. A study of 24 cases. Chirurgie 123:568–571
3. Barber-Westin SD, Noyes FR, McCloskey JW (1999) Rigorous statistical reliability, validity, and responsiveness testing of the Cincinnati knee rating system in 350 subjects with uninjured, injured, or anterior cruciate ligament-reconstructed knees. Am J Sports Med 27:402–416
4. Brittberg M, Lindahl A, Nilsson A, Ohlsson C, Isaksson O, Peterson L (1994) Treatment of deep cartilage defects in the knee with autologous chondrocyte transplantation. N Engl J Med 331:889–895
5. Brittberg M, Tallheden T, Sjogren-Jansson B, Lindahl A, Peterson L (2001) Autologous chondrocytes used for articular cartilage repair: an update. Clin Orthop S337–S348
6. Buckwalter JA, Mankin HJ (1997) Instructional course lectures. The American Academy of Orthopaedic Surgeons – articular cartilage. Part I: Tissue design and chondrocyte-matrix interactions. J Bone Joint Surg-A 79:600–611
7. Buckwalter JA, Mankin HJ (1997) Instructional course lectures, The American Academy of Orthopaedic Surgeons – articular cartilage. Part II: Degeneration and osteoarthrosis, repair, regeneration, and transplantation. J Bone Joint Surg-A 79:612–632

8. Buckwalter JA, Rosenberg LC, Hunziker EB (1990) Articular cartilage: composition, structure, response to injury, and methods of facilitation repair. In: Ewing JW (ed) Articular cartilage and knee joint function. Raven Press, New York, pp19–56
9. Campbell CJ (1969) The healing of cartilage defects. Clin Orthop 64:45–63
10. Erggelet C, Browne JE, Fu F, Mandelbaum BR, Micheli LJ, Mosely JB (2000) Autologous chondrocyte transplantation for treatment of cartilage defects of the knee joint. Clinical results. Zentralbl Chir 125:516–522
11. Erggelet C, Steinwachs MR, Reichelt A (2000) The operative treatment of full thickness cartilage defects in the knee joint with autologous chondrocyte transplantation. Saudi Med 21:715–721
12. Fritsch K-G, Josimovic-Alasevic O (1999) Chondroneogenesis by autologous chondrocyte transplantation (ACT): a cell biological view of consequences for diagnosis and therapy. Arthroskopie 12:43–49
13. Grande DA, Pitman MI, Peterson L, Menche D, Klein M (1989) The repair of experimentally produced defects in rabbit articular cartilage by autologous chondrocyte transplantation. J Orthop Res 7:208–218
14. Grifka J, Anders S, Löhnert J, Baag R, Feldt S (2000) Regeneration of joint cartilage by autologous chondrocyte transplantation. Arthroskopie 13:113–122
15. Hangody L, Kish G, Karpati Z, Udvarhelyi I, Szigeti I, Bely M (1998) Mosaicplasty for the treatment of articular cartilage defects: application in clinical practice. Orthopedics 21:751–756
16. Horas U, Schnettler R, Pelinkovic D, Herr G, Aigner T (2000) Osteochondral transplantation versus autogenous chondrocyte transplantation. A prospective comparative clinical study. Chirurg 71:1090–1097
17. Hunziker EB (1992) Articular cartilage structure in humans and experimental animals. In: Kuettner KE (ed) Articular cartilage and osteoarthritis. Raven Press, New York, pp183–199
18. Löhnert J, Ruhnau K, Gossen A, Bernsmann K, Wiese M (1999) Autologous chondrocyte transplantation (ACT) in the knee joint – first clinical results. Arthroskopie 12:34–42
19. Lysholm J, Gillquist J (1982) Evaluation of knee ligament surgery results with special emphasis on use of a scoring scale. Am J Sports Med 10:150–154
20. Mankin HJ (1982) The response of articular cartilage to mechanical injury. J Bone Joint Surg-A 64:460–466
21. Marshall JL, Fetto JF, Botero PM (1977) Knee ligament injuries: a standardized evaluation method. Clin Orthop115–129
22. Minas T (1998) Chondrocyte implantation in the repair of chondral lesions of the knee: economics and quality of life. Am J Orthop 27:739–744
23. Minas T, Chiu R (2000) Autologous chondrocyte implantation. Am J Knee Surg 13:41–50
24. Peterson L, Brittberg M, Kiviranta I, Akerlund EL, Lindahl A (2002) Autologous chondrocyte transplantation. Biomechanics and long-term durability. Am J Sports Med 30:2–12
25. Peterson L, Minas T, Brittberg M, Nilsson A, Sjogren-Jansson E, Lindahl A (2000) Two- to 9-year outcome after autologous chondrocyte transplantation of the knee. Clin Orthop 374:212–234
26. Poole CA (1997) Articular cartilage chondrons: form, function and failure. J Anat 191 (Pt 1):1–13
27. Scorrano A (1998) Use of resorbable pins to secure the periostal patch in autologous cultured chondrocytes implantation of the knee: initial Italien experience. 2nd Symposium of the International Cartilage Repair Society (ICRS), Boston, USA
28. Wallgren K, Norlin R, Gillquist J (1987) Activity score for the evaluation of orthopedic patients. Proc Scand Orthop Assoc Acta Orthop Scand (Copenhagen) 58:A453

Clinical Results of Autologous Chondrocyte Transplantation (ACT) Using a Collagen Membrane

5

MATTHIAS R. STEINWACHS and PETER C. KREUZ

The treatment of articular cartilage defects is difficult and needs a specialized physician to select the appropriate procedure from a variety of established and new therapeutical approaches. The therapy has to be orientated by the etiology of the cartilage defect. The following categories can be distinguished: degenerative, posttraumatic, inflammatory, metabolic, and vascular toxic cartilage damages. Independent from these categories is the osteochondritis dissecans [22, 51]. The classification of the International Cartilage Repair Society (ICRS) is the standard to describe an articular cartilage defect and is based on the classification of Outerbridge [36]. According to this classification grade III and IV defects have to be treated.

The Structure of Cartilage

The hyaline articular cartilage shows an unique architecture. A superficial tangential zone with approximately 10 to 20% of the whole volume, a middle zone with 40 to 60% volume, and a deep zone with 30% volume can be distinguished. In the superficial zone the cells and the collagen type II fibers are orientated tangentially. In the middle zone the cells are organized in columns and the collagen fibers show a reticular pattern. In the deep zone the cell-fiber mash is attached to the subchondral bone. In this area the fibers have a vertical orientation [20, 23, 34]. The use of MRI has simplified the diagnosis of articular cartilage defects. Today, with the help of cartilage-specific sequences (e.g. 3D-flash sequences) excellent images of the joint cartilage and the subchondral bone are possible [2, 6, 32]. However, regular X-ray to determine the axial and patellar position and ligament instability still has to be performed.

Physiological Cartilage Repair

The therapy of articular cartilage defects is only successful if the concomitant injuries are also treated. In this context, existing varus and valgus deformity and ligament instability have to be considered [7, 10, 28]. The physiological reaction of the organism to a damage of the articular cartilage depends on different factors. The cartilage of growing children has an extremely high regeneration capacity. In contrast, grown man and particularly elderly people have a very low regeneration. Whether this is due to a lower number of MSCs in elderly people is still unclear [8, 9, 49]. The answer of the organism to a damage of the articular cartilage depends on the patient's age and the type and size of the defect.

Chondral and osteochondral defects have to be distinguished. In the surrounding of chondral defects an increase of mitosis and proteoglycan synthesis has been described in animal experiments. However, a cure of these defects has not been observed [12, 15]. The progress of such lesions to osteoarthritis is proven [1, 30, 33, 35]. Similar reactions are detectable in osteochondral defects with an intact subchondral bone plate but healing can also not be expected [31]. As known for chondral lesions the progress to osteoarthritis is also proven. In contrast, osteochondral defects with access to the subchondral bone show limited regeneration. From the bleeding of the subchondral bone a blood clot with a mixture of progenitor cells and fibrin forms, which over time differentiates to a fibrous-like cartilage repair tissue. However, the biomechanical loading capacity of this repair tissue is markedly lower and the collagen composition is not specific for hyaline cartilage. In the long-term regular physiological loading destroys the repair tissue and leads to osteoarthritis [43, 48].

Therapy of Cartilage Defects

The low regeneration capacity makes the refixation of a detached cartilage or cartilage bone fragment with resorbable pins necessary. The indications are flake-fractures and the osteochondritis dissecans. The healing process of these osteochondral lesions is determined by the bone fragment. A horizontal integration of the cartilage fragment into the surrounding intact cartilage can not be expected.

An other procedure is a debridement. This shaving technique combines a lavage, the removal of free bodies and degenerative cartilage fragments, and a limited excision of osteophytes. Studies of Kim et al. [27] have shown that a regeneration of the cartilage is not possible using this technique. Osteoarthritis can not be prevented by washing out degenerative enzymes and detached cartilage pieces. The relatively good clinical results (32 to 74%) at one to four years after surgery [11, 44] could be explained by the removal of active metabolic enzymes from the synovia. Therefore, a debridement is only a palliative method to temporarily relieve patients from pain suffering from an osteoarthritic joint. The use of different laser systems is not recommended because of chondrolysis and osteonecrosis.

The Pridie-drilling [40] is one of the marrow-stimulating techniques. In this procedure holes are drilled into the subchondral bone marrow underneath the regions of the damaged cartilage. The generated blood clot contains progenitor cells and fibrin and differentiates into fibrous cartilage. One of the disadvantages is the heat-induced tissue necrosis at the tip of the drill. The technique is indicated for the treatment of small osteochondral defects and osteochondritis dissecans grade IV. Clinical studies suggest that patients get most benefit from this procedure when axial mal-positioning is corrected as well [47].

In the last years Pridie-drilling was increasingly replaced by microfracturing. The technique is a modification of the Pridie-drilling and thus relays on the same biological principles promoting resurfacing by the formation of fibrocartilaginous repair tissue. The very small micro-holes generated with a special instrument (Chondropick) should be put across the entire cartilage lesion at a distance of 3 to 4 mm and a depth of 4 mm, thus yielding in about 3 to 4 holes per cm^2. Good clinical results with improved joint function and pain reduction during daily activities in 31 to 69% over 3 to 6 years have been reported [37]. The quality of the repair tissue can be improved significantly using CPM after surgery [41].

Another procedure that was first described by Magnuson [29] is the abrasion chondroplasty. This technique gives surgical access to the bone marrow, which together with other vicinal compartments gets stimulated to form a blood clot. The formed tissue is called bioprosthesis, which is fibrous in nature and not durable. The results show that there is a temporary improvement in 60% of the patients [14], but 99% are restricted in their activities of daily life. After 62 months only 12% of the patients are pain free [24–26].

The autologous osteochondral transplantation (OCT or mosaicplasty) is one of the newer procedures in the treatment of cartilage defects. An autologous osteochondral cylinder is harvested from a low weight-bearing area of the joint on transferred into the osteochondral defect. If positioning of the autograft is correct a good surface reconstruction can be expected. Histological analysis revealed a mixture of hyaline (70 to 80%) and fibrous (20 to 30%) cartilage. Symptomatic relief of pain and improvement in joint function have been reported as good and very good (70 to 90%) after one to six years [4, 5, 16, 17]. The procedure is recommended up to a defect size of 3 cm^2. With more cylinders harvested, 5 to 20% of all patients have complaints that may be due to donor site morbidity.

The periosteal transplantation is based on a self-regeneration procedure. The biological background of this principle lies in a cambial layer at the back of the transplanted membrane. This special layer contains progenitor cells that are capable to induce the formation of hyaline-like cartilage. Therefore, the back of the membrane with the cambial layer must be placed into the defect area. The group of Homminga [18] reported about 80% good results using this procedure. Frequently occurring problems are incomplete defect filling and calcification of the periosteal membrane.

For autologous chondrocyte transplantation (ACT) a cartilage biopsy is taken from a non weight-bearing area. The chondrocytes are released and cultured in a special laboratory under GMP-conditions. The quality standards of the ACT and the tissue engineering committee under the patronage of the DGOOC and DGU have to be followed [45]. After expanding, the cells are transported in a special vessel to the hospital. Our own investigations have shown an average cell vitality of more than 84% over a time period of 72 hours after leaving the laboratory (Fig. 5.1A). Required is a continuous cell cooling. Under these conditions 93% of all vital cells are adherent (Fig. 5.1B).

In a second surgical procedure the cartilage defect is prepared. A periosteal flap is harvested and sutured waterproof over the damaged area. The cells are injected underneath the periosteal flap. The cells attach to the subchondral bone and form a cell lawn. They start to produce extracellular matrix and the defect gets filled with a high-quality regenerative tissue. A differentiation of the tissue is possible even without weight-bearing for the first 6 to 8 weeks. CMP for 6 hours a day plays an important role in the nutrition and stimulation of the cells to produce cartilage-like tissue. The use of a periosteal flap revealed in 70 to 90% of all cases good and very good results after two to eleven years [39]. The generated tissue also shows good biome-

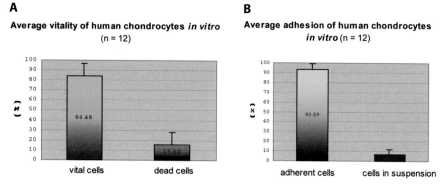

Fig. 5.1A,B. Average cell vitality (A) and cell adhesion (B) of human chondrocytes 24 to 72 hours after leaving the laboratory.

chanical properties. Stiffness tests revealed average solidity values of 3.08 N for healthy hyaline cartilage compared to 2.77 N for the repair tissue after ACT, and 1.23 N for fibrous cartilage after marrow stimulation techniques [38].

Function of the Periosteal Flap

Using periosteum, cartilage formation is promoted by the cambial layer and the injected cells. So far no experimental study has clarified the origin of the cells in the repair tissue. Also, there is no study that has proven a sufficient number of vital cells in the cambial layer of the periosteal flap after cutting the blood supply at the time of harvest. The efficiency of a periosteal graft without ACT could be explained in part because of the bleeding from the subchondral bone and subsequent blood clot formation.

Also, the production of cytokines and growth factors could stimulate the formation of the repair tissue. Our own experiments using periosteal cells have shown a significant synthesis of BMP-2, -4, and -7 but no synthesis of IL-2, IL-6, and IL-8. In 5 to 25% of the cases when a periosteal flap was used a symptomatic hypertrophy has been seen at the repaired surface. Usually the hypertrophic tissue has to be removed in a second intervention. Histologically, the hypertrophic surface is fused to the deep hyaline-like zone [19]. However, especially the superficial tangential zone is of great importance for the biomechanical properties of articular cartilage [50]. The hypertrophic surface leads to an increased friction and progressive fissuration and splitting between the repair tissue and the surrounding healthy cartilage. The consequence is a delamination with loss of the repair tissue. Hypertrophy is not seen in all cases and this is probably due to the fact that the flap is worn out very early after surgery in some cases. A thick periosteal flap harvested from the tibial head comprises a variety of different cell types (e.g. fibroblasts, precursor cells, osteoblasts, and fat cells) that can mix with the transplanted cells and form an inhomogeneous tissue. It is of special importance that fibroblasts have a significant higher proliferation rate compared to chondrocytes.

Freiburg ACT Study
Defect localization

47 Patients with 78 defects

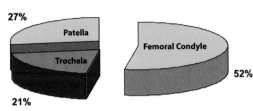

Fig. 5.2.
Distribution of the defect localization in the Freiburg ACT study.

Use of a Collagen Membrane Instead of a Periosteal Flap

The idea that the main function of the periosteal flap is to cover the prepared defect area has inspirited various biotechnology companies to develop different biomaterials for ACT. Collagen is naturally occurring in cartilage and its degradation products are physiological and therefore non-toxic. Due to its good biocompatibility collagen is used in different fields of medicine such as abdominal, plastic or maxillo-facial surgery. The Chondro-Gide® membrane is a bi-layer membrane from porcine collagen type I and III with a smooth outside and a porous inside. The outside has a good mechanical solidity and serves as a barrier, while the inside stimulates through its porous surface the cells to produce cartilage-specific matrix molecules [13]. The membrane is degraded by enzymatic digestion (collagenases). The resulting collagen fragments denature to gelatin and through enzymes such as gelatinase and proteinase to oligopeptides and amino acids.

Animal Experiments Using the Chondro-Gide® Membrane

Osteochondral defects with a diameter of 7 mm were set into the trochlea of the adult sheep. A total of 18 animals were divided into 3 groups. Group I had no treatment, group II was treated with an ACT and a periosteal flap, and in group III an ACT with the Chondro-Gide® membrane was performed. After 1 year the defect was examined histologically and biomechanically. There were no significant differences between group II and III. A complete defect filling could be detected in both groups [42].

Clinical Results

In a clinical study, 125 patients were treated with ACT. Twenty-six% were treated with ACT/periosteal flap and 74% with ACT/Chondro-Gide®. The mean defect size was 4.35 cm² and the mean age 30.9 years. Clinical results after one year turned out to be good or excellent in 89% of all cases. Arthroscopic evaluation after one year revealed in both groups 80.2% ICRS grade I to II cartilage lesions. There were no significant differences in the defect healing and the clinical outcome [3]. Our own clinical studies showed similar results. Cartilage defects in 47 knees with 78 defects were treated either with ACT/periosteal flap (Group I) or with the ACT/Chondro-Gide® membrane (Group II). The mean age was 34.1 years and the mean defect size 5.49 cm². The patients underwent 2.88 surgical interventions before the ACT and were examined clinically with the IKDC-score [21] and radiologically after 3, 6, and 12 months.

In 53% of the cases only one defect and in 47% multiple lesions were treated with ACT. The defects were in 21% at the trochlea, in 27% at the patella, and in 52% at the femoral condyle. The medial femoral condyle was involved most frequently with 85%. In both groups, approximately 80% of the patients had grade IV and 20% grade III lesions. The average value in the ICRS score was 3.81 (SD = 0.39) versus 3.85 (SD = 0.36) in the Chondro-Gide® group. After 6 months the following results were found in the two groups.
- ACT/periosteal flap group: 4.5% grade IV, 53% III, 38% II, and 4.5% grade I.
- ACT/Chondro-Gide® group: 4.8% grade IV, 47.6% III, 47.6% II, and 0% grade I.

The middle score in both groups was 2.57 (SD = 0.66/0.58). After 12 months (Fig. 5.3) the clinical score improved in the ACT/periosteal flap group to 0% grade IV, 30% III, 55% II, and 15% grade I. The ACT/Chondro-Gide® group revealed after 1 year better results: 0% grade IV, 20% III, 40% II, and 40% grade I. The average score was 2.15 (SD = 0.65, periosteal flap) and 1.80 (SD = 0.75, Chondro-Gide®). The study shows a time dependent increase of the IKDC score after 1 year. This could be explained with the biological cartilage remodeling and regeneration after ACT.

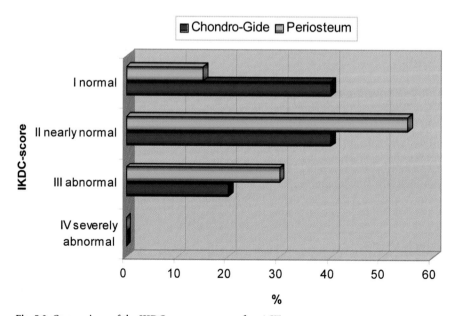

Fig. 5.3. Comparison of the IKDC-score one year after ACT.

Discussion

Considering all the advantages and disadvantages of the different resurfacing methods the surgical therapy of a grade I defect seems not to be necessary. Grade II lesions are usually treated with a arthroscopic debridement. Grade III and IV defects have to be treated. The microfracture technique or the Pridie-drilling can be recommended up to a defect size of 2 cm². Good results can be expected for defect sizes between 1.5 and 3 cm² with osteochondral autografts. Defect sizes between 3 and 10 cm² can be treated successfully only with ACT (Fig. 5.4). The results are good and very good even after follow-up periods of 10 years. There is no other procedure capable to perform an extensive and durable reconstruction of these large cartilage defects. Nevertheless, this procedure has also disadvantages such as hypertrophic changes of the periosteal flap with consecutive pain. The hypertrophic cartilage has to be removed arthroscopically. Another aspect is the remaining superficial unevenness reflecting a not perfect repair of the uppermost cartilage layer. The use of biomaterials may probably solve this problem (Fig. 5.5). However, the effectiveness of such modifications must be tested in clinical studies. The results of our study show that a significant increase (p <0.05) of the clinical scores was observed in both groups. No significant differences could be

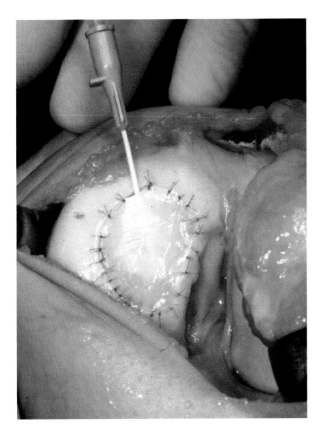

Fig. 5.4.
Collagen membrane
(ChondroGide®, Geistlich
Biomaterials) sutured over
the prepared defect area
instead of a periosteal flap.

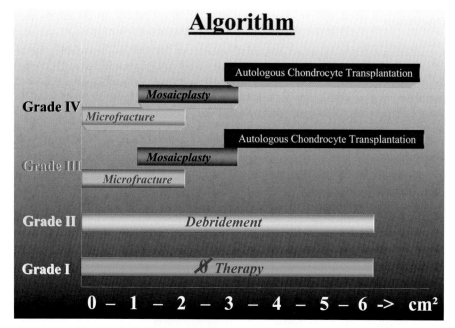

Fig. 5.5. Algorithm for the indication of different surgical techniques in the treatment of cartilage defects.

seen comparing the ACT/periosteal flap group and the ACT/Chondro-Gide® group. High revision rates by periost hypertrophy (5 to 40% in the literature), large interindividual quality differences of the periosteal flap, and an increase of the morbidity by a separate incision are still risk factors in the surgical procedure. According to our clinical results the use of the Chondro-Gide® membrane has the same clinical effectiveness and seems to prevent the complications described above (see Fig. 5.4). The ACT has opened a new dimension in the therapy of cartilage defects. In the treatment of cartilage defects more than 3 cm² the transplantation of chondrocytes is the only procedure to generate a biomechanically high-quality regenerative tissue [46]. The procedure should be performed by specialized surgeons and especially in younger patients with cartilage damages of this size. Future developments will provide a wider application of this technology.

Conclusion

Today, the repair of cartilage defects with hyaline-like repair tissue is possible with 2 methods: the OCT as a one step procedure and the ACT as a two step procedure in the treatment of large isolated defects. For successful ACT a stable bone with an intact tide mark, a high-quality of the chondrocytes, and an exact suture of the flap for closing the bioactive chamber are required. The hypertrophy of the periosteal flap, observed in some cases, can be avoided by the application of biomaterials. The future goal is tissue engineering with mesenchymal stem cells and minimal invasive technologies for a faster rehabilitation and good long-term results in the therapy of articular cartilage repair.

References

1. Aigner T, Glückert K, Mark K (1997) Activation of fibrillar collagen synthesis and phenotypic modulation of chondrocytes in early human osteoarthritic cartilage lesions. Osteoarthritis Cartilage 5:183–185
2. Bachmann G, Heinrichs C, Jürgensen I, Rominger M, Scheiter A, Rau WS (1997) Comparison of different MRT techniques in the diagnosis of degenerative cartilage diseases. In vitro study of 50 joint specimens of the knee at T1.5. Fortschr Rontgenstr 166:429–436
3. Bentley G (2002) Autologous chondrocyte implantation (ACI) in the young adult knee: Clinical, arthroscopic and histological results of 125 patients at 18 month follow up. ICRS, Toronto, Canada
4. Bobic V (1996) Arthroscopic osteochondral autograft transplantation in anterior cruciate ligament reconstruction: a preliminary clinical study. Knee Surg Sports Traumatol Arthrosc 3:262–264
5. Bobic V (1999) Autologe osteochondrale Transplantation zur Behandlung von Gelenkknorpeldefekten. Orthopäde 28:19–25
6. Bohndorf K (1996) Injuries at the articulating surfaces of bone (chondral, osteochondral, subchondral fractures and osteochondrosis dissecans). Eur J Radiol 22:22–29
7. Brittberg M, Lindahl A, Nilsson A, Ohlsson C, Isaksson O, Peterson L (1994) Treatment of deep cartilage defects in the knee with autologous chondrocyte transplantation. N Engl J Med 331:889–895
8. Brittberg M (1997) A critical analysis of cartilage repair. Acta Orthop Scand 68:186–191
9. Caplan AI, Fink DJ, Goto T, Linton AE, Young RG, Wakitani S, Goldberg VM, Haynesworth SE (1993) Mesenchymal stem cells and tissue repair. In: Jackson DW, Arnoczky SP, Frank CB, Woo SL-YY, Simon TM (eds) The anterior cruciate ligament: current and future concepts. Raven Press, New York, pp405–417
10. Erggelet C, Steinwachs M, Reichelt A (1998) Die Behandlung von Gelenkknorpeldefekten. Dtsch Ärztebl 95:1397–1382
11. Friedman MJ, Berasi CC, Fox JM, Del Pizzo W, Snyder SJ, Ferkel RD (1984) Preliminary results with abrasion arthroplasty in the osteoarthritis knee. Clin Orthop 182:200–205
12. Fuller JA, Ghadially FN (1972) Ultrastructural observations on surgically produced partial-thickness defects in articular cartilage. Clin Orthop 86:193–205
13. Fuss M, Ehlers EM et al. (2000) Characteristics of human chondrocytes, osteoblasts and fibroblasts seeded onto a type I/III collagen sponge under different culture conditions. A light scanning and transmission electron microscopy study. Anat Ann 182:303–310
14. Goymann V (1999) Abrasion arthroplasty. Orthopäde 28:11–18
15. Grande DA, Pitman MI, Peterson L, Menche D, Klein M (1989) The repair of experimentally produced defects in rabbit articular cartilage by autologous chondrocyte transplantaion. J Orthop Res 7:208–218
16. Hangody L, Karpati Z (1994) A new surgical treatment of localized cartilaginous defects of the knee. Hungarian J Orthop Trauma 37:237–242
17. Hangody L, Kish G, Karpati Z, Szerb I, Udvarhelyi I (1997) Arthroscopic autogenous osteochondral mosaicplasty for the treatment of femoral condylar articular defects. A preliminary report. Knee Surg Sports Traumatol Arthrose 5:262–267
18. Homminga GN, Bulstra SK, Bouwmeester PS, van der Linden AJ (1990) Perichondral grafting for cartilage lesions of the knee. J Bone Joint Surg-Br 72:1003–1007
19. Horas U, Schnettler R, Perlinkovic D, Herr G, Aigner T (2000) Knorpelknochentransplantation versus autogener Chondrozytentransplantation Chirurg 71:1090–1097

20. Hunziker EB (1992) Articular cartilage structure in humans and experimental animals. In: Kuettner KE, Schleyerbach R, Peyron JG, Articular cartilage and osteoarthritis. Raven Press, New York, 183–199
21. IKDC-Score (1999) International Cartilage Repair Society. ICRS-Newsletter
22. Imhoff A (1991) Kniearthroskopie: Spezielle Diagnostik und Operationstechniken. In: Hempfling H, Burri C (eds) Diagnostische und operative Arthroskopie aller Gelenke. Hans Huber, Bern Stuttgart Toronto, S44–63
23. Jeffery AK, Blunn GW, Archer CW, Bentley G (1991) Three dimensional collagen architecture in bovine articular cartilage. J Bone Joint Surg-Br 73:795–801
24. Johnson LL (1986) Diagnostic and surgical arthroscopy. The knee and other joints, 3nd edn. Mosby, St. Louis
25. Johnson LL (1991) Characteristics of the immediate postarthroscopic blood dot formation in the knee joint. Arthroscopy 7:14–23
26. Johnson LL (1991) Arthroscopic abrasions arthroplasty. In: McGinty JB(ed) Operative Arthroscopy. Raven Press, New York, pp341–360
27. Kim HK, Moran ME, Salter RB (1991) The potential for regeneration of articular cartilage in defects created by chondral shaving and subchondral abrasion. An experimental investigation in rabbits. J Bone Joint Surg-A 73:1301–1315
28. Löhnert J (1999) Autologe Chondrocytentransplantation (ACT) im Kniegelenk. Arthroskopie 12:34–42
29. Magnuson PB (1941) Joint debridement surgical treatment of degenerative arthritis. Surg Gynecol Obstet 73:1–9
30. Maletius W, Aigner T (1999) Morphologie und Molekularpathologie der Osteoarthrose – Relevanz für Pathogenese und Diagnostik. Arthroskopie 12:3–8
31. Mankin HJ (1982) The response of articular cartilage to mechanical injury. J Bone Joint Surg-A 64:460–466
32. McCauley T, Disler D (1998) MRI of articular cartilage. Radiology 209:629–640
33. Messner K, Maletius W (1996) The long-term prognosis for severe damage of the weight-bearing cartilage in the knee. Acta Orthop Scand 67:165–168
34. Metz J (2001) Makroskopie, Histologie und Zellbiologie des Gelenkknorpels. In: Erggelet C, Steinwachs M (eds) Gelenkknorpeldefekte. Steinkopff, Darmstadt, S3–13
35. Mohr W (1998) Morphogenese der Osteoarthrose. Arthroskopie 6:195–200
36. Outerbridge RE (1961) The etiology of chondromalacia patellae. J Bone Joint Surg-Br 43:752–757
37. Pässler HH (2001) Knochenmarkstimulierende Techniken – Mikrofracture. In: Erggelet C, Steinwachs M (eds) Gelenkknorpeldefekte. Steinkopff, Darmstadt, S83–92
38. Peterson L (1998) Autologous chondrocyte transplantation: 2–10 year follow-up in 219 patients. Annual Meeting of the American Academy of Orthopaedic Surgeons, New Orleans, March 21, 1998
39. Peterson L, Brittberg M, Kiviranta I, Akerlund EL, Lindahl A (2002) Autologous chondrocyte transplantation, biomechanics and long-term durability. Am J Sports Med 30:2–12
40. Pridie KH (1959) A method of resurfacing osteoarthritic knee joints. J Bone Joint Surg-Br 41:618–619
41. Rodrigo JJ, Steadman JR, Silliman JF, Fulstone HA (1994) Improvement in full-thickness chondral defect healing in the human knee after debridement and microfracture using continuous passive motion. Am J Knee Surg 7:109–116
42. Russlies et al. (2002) Histological and biomechanical results of 3 different cartilage repair technique in a sheep model. ICRS 2002, Toronto
43. Shapiro F, Koide S, Glimcher MJ (1993) Cell origin and differentiation in the repair of full-thickness defects of articular cartilage. J Bone Joint Surg-A 75:532–553
44. Sprague NF 3rd (1981) Arthroscopic debridement for regeneration knee joint disease. Clin Orthop 160:118–123
45. Stellungnahme der Arbeitgemeinschaft – Autologe Chondrozyten-Transplantation (ACT) und Tissue Engineering – unter Schirmherrschaft der DGU und DGOOC (2002) Z Orthop 140:132–137

46. Steinwachs MR, Erggelet C, Lahm A, Guhlke-Steinwachs U (1999) Clinical and cell biology aspects of autologous chondrocytes transplantation. Unfallchirurg 102:855–860
47. Tippet JW (1996) Articular cartilage drilling and osteotomy in ostoarthritis of the knee. In: McGinty JB, Caspari RB, Jackson RW, Poehling GG (eds) Operative arthroscopy, 2nd edn. Raven Press, Philadelphia, New York, pp411–426
48. Wakitani S, Goto T, Pineda SJ, Young RG, Mansour JM, Caplan AI, Goldberg VM (1994) Mesenchymal cell-based repair of large, full-thickness defects of articular cartilage. J Bone Joint Surg-A 76:579–592
49. Wirth CJ, Rudert M (1996) Techniques of cartilage growth enhancement: a review of the literature. J Arthrosc Rel Surg 12:300–308
50. Wong M, Wuetherich P, Buschmann M, Eggli P, Hunziker EB (1997) Chondrocyte biosynthesis correlates with local tissue strain in statically compressed adult articular cartilage. J Orthop Res 15:189–196
51. Zollinger H (1977) Indikation und Aussage der Gelenkendoskopie bei der Chondropathia patellae. Z Orthop (abstract) 115:617

Treatment of Chondral Defects by Matrix-Guided Autologous Chondrocyte Implantation (MACI)*

6

Erhan Basad, Henning Stürz and Jürgen Steinmeyer

Introduction

Articular cartilage is not capable of self-repair. Traumatic damages are one of the most common causes of the premature onset of osteoarthritis. Cartilage is avascular and therefore regeneration is different compared to wound healing in tissues with an extensive blood supply [6, 9]. Currently, stimulating (microfracture, Pridie-drilling, and abrasion arthroplasty) and reparative techniques (mosaicplasty, ACT, MACI, perichondrium- and periosteal flap transplantation) are available for surgical treatment of cartilage defects. Using stimulating techniques a fibrocartilage is formed. In these techniques the subchondral bone plate in the area of the cartilage defect has to be penetrated and mesenchymal progenitor cells are recruited from the bone marrow.

During mosaicplasty [5, 8] autologous osteochondral cylinders are inserted into the drilled defect. Limitations of this method are restricted availability of cylinders, the fact that the surface of the joint is incompletely restored (cobblestone phenomenon), and donor site morbidity. Methods using the implantation of autologous chondrocytes grown *in vitro* are currently under clinical investigation. Accordingly, autologous chondrocyte transplantation (ACT) [4, 15] with the formation of hyaline-like cartilage is used more and more frequently. Aims of this new therapeutic concept are the filling of the defect with hyaline cartilage, the restoration of the joint surface, the painless and unrestricted mobility of the joint, and the prevention of progressive degeneration of the joint.

The combination of cell transplantation and tissue engineering techniques offers new therapeutical possibilities, which are currently undergoing clinical trials. Matrix-guided autologous chondrocyte transplantation (MACI) [2] is one of those. The special feature in this new procedure is the use of a collagen type I/II-membrane, which is loaded with chondrocytes *in vitro* (1×10^6 cells per cm^2) and subsequently implanted. There are two reasons for not using collagen type II, which is the dominant collagen in the hyaline articular cartilage for the production of the collagen membrane:

1. Injection of collagen type II into a joint with cartilage damage may lead to an increase in enzymatic break down [14].
2. Compared to collagen type I and III, collagen type II is difficult to process.

* This work was supported by Verigen AG

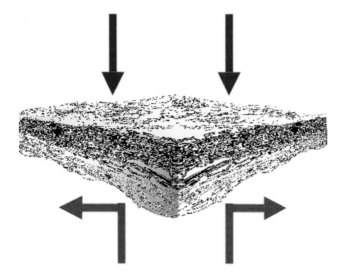

Fig. 6.1.
Collagen type I/III-matrix with the cell permeable (*blue*) and the cell occlusive (*red*) surface. The cell permeable surface is fixed to the subchondral bone plate with fibrin glue.

In vitro experiments have shown that chondrocytes can attach to a collagen type I/III-matrix and re-differentiate [7, 16]. The collagen matrix loaded with chondrocytes is implanted in a second operation. A particular advantage is that the membrane is fixed using a very small amount of fibrin glue, replacing earlier techniques where the membrane was fixed by suturing. In this respect, MACI represents a more simple surgical technique compared to ACT. The three-dimensional network of the support material promotes the re-differentiation and attachment of the chondrocytes [7]. The collagen type I/III-matrix (Fig. 6.1) gets remodeled within a few months and replaced by the extracellular matrix of the regenerate [20].

Choosing a surgical technique for the treatment of a cartilage lesions is not easy because no comparative studies have been carried out so far. Thus, the aim of this study was to compare MACI and microfracturing using clinical tests. The patients were followed-up for up to 1 year using symptomevaluating scores.

Materials and Methods

The inclusion criteria for the study were:
- age 18 to 50 years,
- isolated chondral or osteochondral defect (2 cm² to 10 cm²),
- condylar and/or retropatellar localization.

The exclusion criteria for the study were:
- unstable knee joint,
- total meniscectomy,
- varus or valgus deformity,
- other joint or skeletal diseases (e.g. osteonecrosis, chondrocalcinosis, osteoarthritis, and rheumatoid arthritis),
- allergies to gentamycine, bovine or porcine products,

- pregnancy,
- overweight (BMI >30).

For the determination of knee function the following scores were used:

- Meyers score,
- Tegner-Lysholm score,
- Lysholm-Gilquist score,
- ICRS classification.

All surgery and postoperative examinations were carried out by the same investigator. All patients was examined at least 6 or 7 times within the first year (Table 6.1):

The surgical procedure and cell culture technique in the MACI group was as follows:

1. *First surgery*: Drawing of blood to obtain autologous serum. Arthroscopic harvest of an approximately 2 mm³ cartilage biopsy from the edge of the intercondylar notch. Packaging and sending the cartilage biopsy in sterile medium to the cell culture laboratory at Verigen Transplantation Service International AG (Leverkusen, Germany) according to safety and quality requirements of GMP directives (Good Manufacturing Practices).

2. *In vitro processing*: Mechanical grinding and washing of the cartilage pieces in PBS (phosphate buffered saline). Incubation in enzyme containing medium (collagenase and dispase) at 37 °C for 2 to 4 hours to release chondrocytes. Culture of the cells at 37 °C with medium and autologous serum. Changing the medium at several time points until at least 1×10^6 chondrocytes were available. Loading of a collagen type I/III-membrane with the cultured cells. Viability (minimum 85% living cells), cell density per cm² of the membrane (approximately $1\times10^6/cm^2$), and sterility of the implant were tested (Fig. 6.2).

3. *Second surgery:* Mini-arthrotomy and debridement of the defect with trimming the surrounding healthy cartilage. It is essential that the subchondral bone plate is not damaged during the debridement of the defect area. However, should bleeding occur this can be stopped by using epinephrine (Suprarenin®). Exact determination of the dimensions of the defect was performed by impression onto a piece of aluminum foil. The collagen matrix loaded with chondrocytes was cut and placed into the defect area and fixed with fibrin glue (Tissucol®, Baxter AG, Munich) (Fig. 6.3). During hardening of the fibrin adhesive the knee was brought in extension. Consequently, the opposing surface (tibia concavity) gives an exact impression. Stability of the implant was tested during surgery by movement of the knee joint. Bleeding was stopped carefully because no intraarticular drain was used. A sterile wound dressing was applied and the leg initially set at 10° flexion in a dorsal cast.

4. *Postsurgical treatment:* Postsurgical treatment started with a one week immobilization, followed by mobilization with 10 kg weight-bearing (floor contact) for 8 to 12 weeks. The CPM was used after the first week. During the first 6 weeks ROM was restricted depending on the location of the defect from 30° to 90° flexion, using a knee brace (Collamed II®, Medi Bayreuth GmbH, Bayreuth, Germany).

In the control group microfracturing was performed by a single arthroscopic operation in a randomized manner (see Table 6.1). Postoperative treatment was 6 weeks partial weight-bearing and CPM from the 2nd to the 6th week.

Table 6.1. Description of the study design

	Inclusion	1st surgery	2nd surgery	Rehabili-tation	Follow-up	Follow-up	Follow-up
MACI	Random-ized	Arthoscopy + biopsy	MACI	1st to 6th week	3 months	6 months	12 months
MFX	Random-ized	Arthoscopy + MFX	n/n	2nd to 6th week	3 months	6 months	12 months

n/n not necessary, *MFX* microfraturing.

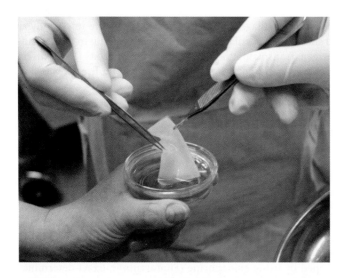

Fig. 6.2.
The collagen matrix loaded with chondrocytes before implantation. The implant is surrounded by a red-coloured nutrition medium during transportation.

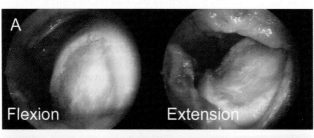

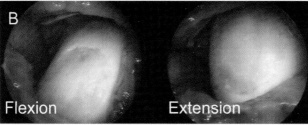

Fig. 6.3A,B.
(**A**) Debridement of the chondral defect without injuring the subchondral plate. (**B**) Defect after fixation of the implant with fibrin glue.

Results

Today, approximately 800 patients have been treated with MACI worldwide. Experience with MACI has been gained in the last 2 years. Between July 2000 and August 2002, 30 patients (18 MACI and 12 microfracturing) were treated in a randomized, prospective and controlled study. The mean age was 34.6 years, the mean height 179.7 cm (SD = 13.1), and the mean weight 78.8 kg (SD = 14.1). By August 2002 the results of 6 patients for a follow-up of 1 year were available.

The Meyers score [13] evaluates criteria for pain, walking and range of motion with a maximum of 18 points. According to Meyers et al. the points are assessed as followed:

- 18 points for excellent,
- 15 to 17 for good,
- 12 to 15 for fair,
- below 12 for bad.

The results for the MACI showed an improvement of 7 points whereas for microfracturing the score raised only 1 point (Fig. 6.4).

The Lysholm and Gillquist score [12] was originally developed for the assessment of knee instability. Pain and instability covers 30% of the criteria. Limping, crutches, ability to squat down, and muscle circumference are counting with 5% each. Stair climbing and swelling is assessed with 10%. A patient without symptoms can reach the maximum of 100 points. The MACI group showed 1 year after surgery an improvement of 52 points, whereas the score of the microfracturing group increased by 16 points (Fig. 6.5).

In 1985 Tegner and Lysholm [19] published an evaluation protocol where the activity of the patient is rationed in 11 grades (0 to 10). Level 10 is only achieved by national and international athletes, while patients with level 0 are serious disabled because of their knee problems. The MACI group showed an improvement of 1.7 points. The microfracturing group with –0.4 points showed a minimal decrease in the activity score (Fig. 6.6).

The advanced International Knee Documentation Committee (IKDC) score, which was released by the International Cartilage Research Society (ICRS) is divided into a surgeons and a patients form. The following forms were used with little modifications:

1. IKDC subjective knee evaluation form 2000 (patient)
2. ICRS knee history registration previous surgery (surgeon)
3. IKDC knee examination form 2000 (surgeon)

The calculated classification has 4 grades. The discomfort of the patient impairs with increasing of the grade. Table 6.2 shows that both surgical techniques can improve the score by reducing discomfort.

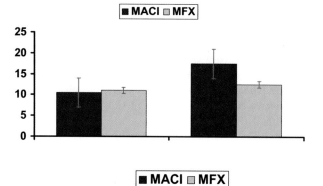

Fig. 6.4.
The Meyers score of patients treated either with MACI of MFX (= microfracturing) before and one year after surgery. Data are expressed as mean values ± SD (n = 6).

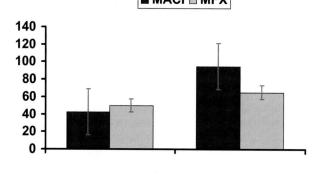

Fig. 6.5.
The Lysholm-Gillquist score of patients treated either with MACI or MFX (= microfracturing) before and one year after surgery. Data are expressed as mean values ± SD (n = 6).

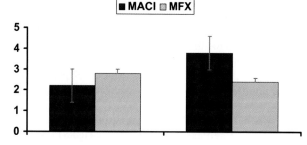

Fig. 6.6.
The Tegner-Lysholm score of patients treated either with MACI or MFX (= microfracturing) before and one year after surgery. Data are expressed as mean values ± SD (n = 6).

Table 6.2. The IKDC score of patients treated either with MACI or MFX before and one year after surgery (n = 6)

IKDC Score	Grade I [%]	Grade II [%]	Grade III [%]	Grade IV [%]	n.d. [%]
Before surgery:					
MACI	0.0	0.0	50.0	50.0	0.0
MFX	0.0	0.0	60.0	20.0	20.0
1 year after surgery:					
MACI	50.0	33.3	16.7	0.0	0.0
MFX	40.0	20.0	20.0	0.0	20.0

n.d. not determined.

Discussion

Microfracturing is an established and cost effective procedure resulting in the formation of fibrous cartilage and providing good results in the mid-term [18]. It is therefore necessary that expensive cell-based procedures prove their superiority over microfracturing in the form of prospective, controlled, and randomized studies. Since the introduction of ACT, numerous research groups have experimentally and clinically worked with cell-based therapy of cartilage defects. Already in clinical trials the first results have been encouraging with good to excellent results [1, 15].

Problems and limitations of ACT must also be mentioned. Human chondrocytes de-differentiate in monolayer cultures, with the result that they no longer differ form fibroblasts after a few weeks [17]. It has been shown that after a 42-day culture period mRNA for collagen type II and chondromodulin is no longer expressed. However, tests for cartilage unspecific collagen types I and III were positive. Histomorphological analysis of the cartilage regenerate showed clear differences compared to the surrounding cartilage 12 months after ACT, in some cases with formation of fibrous cartilage [10, 11]. The bonding of the ACT regenerate to the surrounding cartilage and the subchondral bone plate is often unsatisfactory. In addition, the typical morphological appearance such as rooting of the extracellular matrix into the subchondral bone plate and the arcade-like alignment of the collagen fibers is lacking [3].

The role of the periosteal flap in ACT is of current research interest. Adhesions in the joint may result from hypertrophic tissue proliferation of the periosteal flap. Damage to adjoining areas of cartilage due to suturing of the periosteal flap has also been described [1, 17]. High technical challenges are facing the surgeon regarding the fixation and sealing of the periosteal flap. If there is a lack of a cartilage rim, e.g. if the defect is close to the intercondylar notch, ACT reaches its limitations.

In vitro and *in vivo* experiments with the chondrocyte-loaded collagen type I/III-matrix have already shown that the chondrocytes proliferate and are able to synthesize cartilage-specific molecules [7, 16]. Advantages of MACI over ACT are the simplified surgical technique and the considerable reduction of time required for surgery (approximately 45 min). The removal of the periosteal flap and the suturing of the transplant are not needed and a smaller skin cut can be made. In addition, the complex three-dimensional convex (or concave) surface of the femoral condyle or the patella can more easily recreated using the moldable collagen carrier.

In contrast to ACT, MACI represents a simplified surgical technique for successful remodeling of the articular cartilage surface. Our good to very good clinical results are promising. Further tests with a larger number of patients and covering a longer time period are necessary and are currently carried out. A correct anatomical axis and ligament stability must be present before MACI can be performed. With ACT and MACI cell-based surgical procedures with promising clinical results are available for the orthopaedic surgeon.

References

1. Anders S, Schaumburger J, Grifka J (2001) Intraartikuläre operative Maßnahmen bei Arthrose. Orthopäde 30:866–880
2. Behrens P, Ehlers EM, Kochermann KU, Rohwedel J, Russlies M, Plotz W (1999) New therapy procedure for localized cartilage defects. Encouraging results with autologous chondrocyte implantation. MMW Fortschr Med 141:49–51
3. Breinan HA, Minas T, Hsu HP, Nehrer S, Sledge CB, Spector M(1997) Effect of cultured autologous chondrocytes on repair of chondral defects in a canine model. J Bone Joint Surg-A 79:1439–1451
4. Brittberg M, Lindahl A, Nilsson A, Ohlsson C, Isaksson O, Peterson L (1994) Treatment of deep cartilage defects in the knee with autologous chondrocyte transplantation. N Engl J Med 331:889–895
5. Burkart AC, Schoettle PB, Imhoff AB (2001) Operative Therapiemöglichkeiten des Knorpelschadens. Unfallchirurg 104:798–807
6. Curl WW, Krome J, Gordon ES, Rushing J, Smith BP, Poehling GG (1997) Cartilage injuries: a review of 31,516 knee arthroscopies. Arthroscopy 4:456–460
7. Fuss M, Ehlers EM, Russlies M, Rohwedel J, Behrens P (2000) Characteristics of human chondrocytes, osteoblasts and fibroblasts seeded onto a type I/III collagen sponge under different culture conditions. A light, scanning and transmission electron microscopy study. Anat Anz 182:303–310
8. Hangody L, Feczko P, Bartha L, Bodo G, Kish G (2001) Mosaicplasty for the treatment of articular defects of the knee and ankle. Clin Orthop 391 [Suppl]:S328–336
9. Hauselmann HJ, Hunziker EB (1997) Lesions of articular cartilage and their treatment. Schweiz Med Wochenschr 127:1911–1924
10. Hunziker EB (2002) Articular cartilage repair: basic science and clinical progress. A review of the current status and prospects. Osteoarthritis Cartilage 10:432–463
11. Hunziker EB, Quinn TM, Hauselmann HJ (2002) Quantitative structural organization of normal adult human articular cartilage. Osteoarthritis Cartilage 10:564–572
12. Lysholm J, Gillquist J (1982) Evaluation of knee ligament surgery results with special emphasis on use of a scoring scale. Am J Sports Med 10:150–154
13. Meyers MH, Akerson W, Convery FR (1989) Resurfacing of the knee with fresh osteochondral allograft. J Bone Joint Surg-A 71:704–713
14. Myers LK, Rosloniec EF, Cremer MA, Kang AH (1997) Collagen-induced arthritis, an animal model of autoimmunity. Life Sci 61:1861–1878
15. Peterson L, Brittberg M, Kiviranta I, Akerlund EL, Lindahl A (2002) Autologous chondrocyte transplantation. Biomechanics and long-term durability. Am J Sports Med 30:2–12
16. Russlies M, Behrens P, Wunsch L, Gille J, Ehlers EM (2002) A cell-seeded biocomposite for cartilage repair. Ann Anat 184:317–323
17. Schnabel M, Marlovits S, Eckhoff G, Fichtel I, Gotzen L, Vecsei V, Schlegel J (2002) Dedifferentiation-associated changes in morphology and gene expression in primary human articular chondrocytes in cell culture. Osteoarthritis Cartilage 10:62–70
18. Steadman JR, Rodkey WG, Briggs KK (2002) Microfracture to treat full-thickness chondral defects: surgical technique, rehabilitation, and outcomes. J Knee Surg 15:170–176
19. Tegner Y, Lysholm J (1985) Rating systems in the evaluation of knee ligament injuries. Clin Orthop 198:42–49
20. Zheng M (2002) Biodegradable collagene membrane is more effective then periosteal flap in ACI: a rabbit study. ICRS meeting, Toronto

CHAPTER 7

Transplantation of Osteochondral Autografts   7

ANDREAS WERNER and JÜRGEN ARNOLD

Introduction

Articular cartilage lesions in the adult have no potential for a *restitutio ad integrum* [6, 24]. Natural regeneration of the joint surface is limited to a repair cartilage with a high rate of collagen type I and low biomechanical strength compared to normal hyaline cartilage [6]. This repair tissue is at a high risk for degeneration with new clinical symptoms [11, 26]. Efficient treatment of symptomatic full-thickness cartilage defects is still a challenge for the surgeon. Several techniques are currently used: debridement of the defect alone, initiation of mesenchymal cell migration from the subchondral bone to build a repair tissue by microfracturing [34], drilling [29], abrasion [21], and transplantation of cultured autologous chondrocytes [28]. Transplantation of osteochondral grafts is currently the only technique to fill a joint surface defect with hyaline cartilage.

In 1964 Wagner [35] reported about autologous osteochondral transplantation (OCT) for the treatment of osteochondritis dissecans in the knee. Later, other authors like Yamashita et al. [38] reported about similar techniques. Also, osteochondral allografts were used [9] but because of the possible risk of disease transmission, tissue metaplasia and questionable viability of the grafts, most authors turned to autologous transplantation. In 1993, Matsusue et al. [25] published the first report about arthroscopic osteochondral transplanation. This was later repopularized by Bobic [4]. Hangody et al. [12–14] introduced the "mosaicplasty" using several small transplants to cover a defect. In 1999, Imhoff et al. [19] presented the transfer of the posterior femoral condyle as a salvage procedure in major defects. Today osteochondral transplantation is used not only in the knee but also in other joints such as the ankle, the elbow, and shoulder [3, 16, 18].

Indications for Osteochondral Transplantation

Different factors are of relevance for the choice of the treatment for osteochondral lesions: etiology of the defect, size and depth of the lesion, localization, age of the patient, and concomitant pathology as joint instability, varus/valgus deformities or systemic diseases like rheumatoid arthritis.

Accepted indications for osteochondral transplantation are deep focal chondral or osteochondral defects of the femoral condyles, the trochlea, the patella, and the talus.

Relative indications include defects in other joints such as the shoulder, the elbow or the hip [18]. Today, also larger defects in the knee or beginning osteoarthritis in young patients are treated with osteochondral transplants as joint preserving salvage procedures [23].

Indications for Autologous Osteochondral Transplantation (modified from [18])

- Focal osteochondral lesions > 1 to 9 cm² (ICRS grade 4) in the weight-bearing area of the femoral condyle, patella/trochlea and talus edge
- Local cartilaginous lesions (Outerbridge grade 3 and 4, ICRS grade 2 and 3) > 1 to 9 cm² in the weight-bearing area of the femoral condyle, patella/trochlea and talus edge
- Osteochondritis dissecans (grade 3 and 4) and local osteonecrosis > 1 to 9 cm² in the weight-bearing area of the femoral condyle, patella/trochlea and talus edge
- Relative: similar lesions of the shoulder, elbow and hip, local osteonecrosis, beginning osteoarthritis in young patients

---

Contraindications are larger defects, infection or aseptic arthritis, e.g. rheumatoid arthritis, corresponding ("kissing") defects, bad quality of the surrounding bone, and general osteoarthritis. Open epiphyses in the adolescent are not a contraindication as long as they remain untouched by the procedure. Concomitant joint pathologies like cruciate ligament insufficiency, varus or valgus deformities or patella mal-tracking have to be corrected with or before the osteochondral transplantation.

General Technique of Osteochondral Autograft Transplantation

Today, different systems and instruments are available for this procedure. In general, intact osteochondral cylinders are harvested from a donor site and transplanted into pre-drilled holes in the defect area. The donor grafts have a slightly bigger diameter to allow press fit implantation. Grafts can be harvested using tubular hollow chisels, e.g. the OATS©-System (Arthrex, Naples, Florida, USA) or with wet grinding systems like the diamond coated SDI©-system (medArtis, Munich, Germany). It is important to identify the identical surface anatomy of the defect when choosing the donor graft. Usually, the tool for harvesting the cylinder must be inserted in perpendicular direction to the donor surface, otherwise the graft might not fit into the recipient hole or the cartilage layer might shear off. Only if, like e.g. for the talus, the insertion is better performed in an oblique fashion, we adapt this to the procedure. Most instruments allow obtaining grafts from 5 to 11 mm in diameter, while Hangody et al. [12–14] used also smaller grafts down to 2.7 mm. The length of the osteochondral graft should be at least 13 to 15 mm, while for deeper osseous defects it can easily be extended to 25 mm. Depending of the diameter of the defect, it can be restored with only one bigger transplant or with several smaller grafts. With his "mosaicplasty", Hangody [12, 13, 16] was able to cover 60% to 90% of a given defect with several smaller grafts. In this technique, the remaining defect area between the transplanted cylinders is not covered with hyaline cartilage, but supposed to be filled with fibrocartilage. Also, grafts can be implanted in a more overlapping "puzzle-technique" [4, 8, 17], which allows (almost) complete restoration of the joint surface. For this technique, the grafts usually have a larger diameter than for the mosaicplasty. Theoretically, the integration of the grafts in the surrounding joint surface in the latter technique reduce shear stresses on the graft surface compared to the mosaicplasty and should allow early weight-bearing. On the other hand, restoration of the shape of the joint surface might better be accomplished with several smaller grafts (Fig. 7.1 and 7.2).

Commonly used donor sites are the borders of the lateral or medial femoral condyle above the level of the *linea terminalis* or the edges of the intercondylar notch. Also, the posterior aspect of the femoral condyles can be used. [4, 12, 13, 18, 27, 35, 38]. Simonian [33] showed that the proximal aspect of the lateral femoral condyle and the medial aspect of the notch had the lowest contact pressures between 0 and 110° knee flexion. Still, there was no area in the knee without any contact pressure. His concerns lead other authors to evaluate further potential autologous donor sites. For OCT of the talus, Sammarco et al. [30] recently described the talar articular facet as a useful donor region.

The donor defects are usually filled with bone from the osteochondral cylinder taken from the defect zone, eventually additionally with collagen membranes. The defects are normally filled by bone and fibrocartilage after 3 months, which reach the level of the surrounding cartilage after 1 year [4]. Alternatively, periosteum-covered plugs harvested from the iliac crest [17] or synthetic material such as tricalcium phosphate or hydroxyapatite can be used to fill the donor site defect.

Osteochondral allografts as fresh or frozen tissue can be transplanted as cylindrical grafts like in the autologous techniques or they can be adapted to the original defect geometry.

Osteochondral transplantation can be performed as an arthroscopic, mini-open or conventional open procedure. Arthroscopy is suitable only for smaller defects of the weight-bearing area of the femoral condyles, while other locations are usually treated by an open procedure. Especially in patients with a tight patellofemoral articulation, a lateral release can be added to reduce the contact pressure at the femoral harvest site after autologous transfer from the lateral condyle.

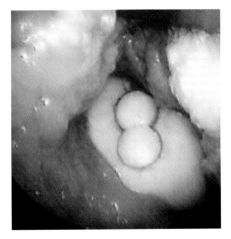

Fig. 7.1. Intra-operative view of autologous OCT in the knee (femoral condyle).

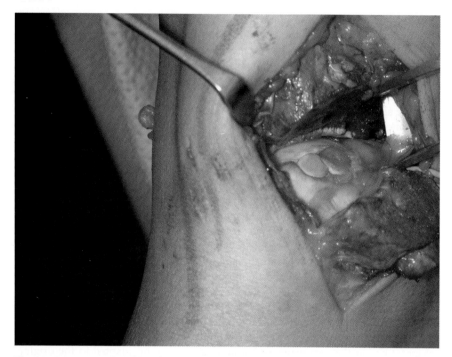

Fig. 7.2. Intra-operative view of autologous OCT in the talus (with osteotomy of the medial malleolus).

Results of Osteochondral Transplantation

Basic Science Studies

Animal studies showed that a complete osseous ingrowth of the graft below the tide mark could be achieved, while there was no real integration at the level of the cartilage layer [8, 12, 16, 32]. Hangody et al. [12, 16] saw a fibrocartilaginous scar tissue between graft and surrounding tissue. This was supported by Siebert et al. [32]. Biopsies taken during second look arthroscopy demonstrated survival of the chondrocytes and a remaining hyaline-type of cartilage [4, 16].

Results of Autolgous Osteochondral Transplantation in the Knee

In 1972, Wagner [36] already presented good results in 20 of 26 patients with autologous osteochondral transplantation and a 9-year follow-up. Laprell and Petersen [22] saw 12 of 29 normal and 14 of 29 almost normal knees according to the ICSS scale after 6 to 12 years following autologous OCT. Outerbridge et al. [27] found improved function and reduced pain 6.5 years after transplantation of autologous patella grafts into defects of the femoral condyles. Recently, Hangody et al. [16] reported good results in 91% of 126 patients after mosaicplasty with a minimum follow-up of 3 years. Jakob et al. [20] reported improved knee function in 92% of 52 patients after 37 (24–56) months. Burkart et al. [7] found an average of 91 points in the Lysholm score in 156 patients 12 to 52 months after OCT using the OATS©-technique. Attmanspacher et al. [2] treated 27 patients with the same system and an average defect diameter of 15 mm. Short term results were good with a Lysolm Score of 88 (78 to 93) points (Table 7.1).

Results of Autologous Osteochondral Transplantation in the Talus

Recent experience with autologous osteochondral transplantation in the talus demonstrated results comparable to the knee joint after mid-term follow-up. Hangody [15] reported good and excellent results in 34 of 36 patients after 2 to 7 years. Gautier et al. [10] saw good to excellent results in 11 of 11 patients after a mean follow-up of 2 years, Al-Shaikh et al. [1] found an average postoperative AOFAS ankle score of 88 (60 to 100) in a group of 19 patients after 18 (12 to 30) months. Schoettle et al. [31] reported an average Lysholm and Bruns score of 92 points after 6 to 42 months in 39 patients. Baltzer et al. [3] found 15 of 16 patients symptom free after 6 months after OCT for posttraumatic lesions or OCD of the talus. Interestingly, none of the authors reported about problems with the knee at the donor site, except 2 patients with mild knee pain in Al-Shaik´s study [1]. Sammarco [30] used local grafts from the medial or lateral articular facet on the same side of the lesion. All 12 patients in his study had significant improvement of symptoms and an AOFAS score of 90.8 points after 25 months follow-up (Table 7.2).

Table 7.1. Results of autologous OCT in the knee

Author	Patients [n]	Follow-up [months]	Results
Bobic	12	24	10/12 good/excellent
Burkart	156	21 (12–52)	Lysholm 58:91 P
Hangody	126	36 (min)	91% good/excellent
Jakob	52	24–56	92% improved

Table 7.2. Results of autologous OCT in the talus

Author	Donor site	Patients [n]	Follow up [months]	Results
Al-Shaikh	Knee	19	12 to 30	17/19 good/excellent
Gaultier	Knee	11	24	11/11 good/excellent
Hangody	Knee	36	50 (24 to 84)	34/36 good/excellent
Sammarco	Talus	12	25	12/12 good/excellent
Schoettle	Knee	39	19.6 (6 to 42)	Lysholm 62:92 P

Technical Pitfalls and Complications of Osteochondral Transplantation

Technical Pitfalls

There are some technical considerations in OCT. Inadequate length of the cylinder can be corrected by replanting cancellous bone from the recipient cylinder (too short) or shortening the graft (too long). High impacting forces on the graft should be avoided not to destroy its cartilage layer. Graft length must be at least 10 mm for secure press fit fixation. Inadequate positioning of the graft should be avoided, first by proper selection of the harvest site according to the required contour of the defect area, and then by careful manipulation during insertion. Finally, fractures of the donating condyle are reported [4].

Postoperative Complications

Postoperative complications of OCT are unspecific problems like hemarthroses, joint effusions or persistent swelling [4, 5, 16]. The rates reported are comparable to other major joint surgeries. Method-specific complications are pain at the donor site, mostly appearing as patellofemoral pain, secondary graft subsidence, loose bodies, and avascular necrosis after harvesting too many grafts from one site [4]. Incongruency of the corresponding joint surfaces by different curvatures of donor and recipient, or insufficient reconstruction of the level of the subchondral bone, may lead to early degeneration of the transplant [18]. Hangody reported that donor site problems were only transient. In patients, in whom the knee served only for procurement of the osteochondral plugs, knee complaints resolved in 95% after 6 weeks and in 98% after 1 year. Imhoff and Oettl [18] found transient retropatellar pain in 20% of their patients. On the other hand, Wirth et al. [37] reported that after 3.7 years all donor site condyles showed progression of a pre-existing osteoarthritis.

Conclusion

Today, OCT is the only technique to replace a destroyed articular surface by real hyaline cartilage, with good mid-term results in the literature. Existing instruments for autologous OCT allow adequate repair of defects up to 20 to 25 mm in diameter. Larger defects may be treated as a salvage procedure, but donor tissue is limited. Allograft transplantation is possible, but includes the risk of disease transmission or limited viability of the graft. Intra-operative pitfalls have to be considered. The question of potential donorsite morbidity appears to be of little clinical relevance, but is certainly not definitively answered yet.

References

1. Al-Shaikh RA, Chou LB, Mann JA, Dreeben SM, Prieskorn D (2002) Autologous osteochondral grafting for talar cartilage defects. Foot Ankle Int 23:381–389
2. Attmanspacher W, Dittrich V, Stedtfeld HW (2000) Klinische Erfahrungen und kurzfristige Ergebnisse mit OATS. Arthroskopie 13:103–108
3. Baltzer AW, Becker C, Liebau C, Krauspe R, Merk HR (2000) Knorpel-Knochen-Transplantation am oberen Sprunggelenk. Arthroskopie 13:109–112
4. Bobic V (1999) Die Verwendung von autologen Knochen-Knorpel-Transplantaten in der Behandlung von Gelenkknorpelläsionen. Orthopäde 28:19–25
5. Boes L, Ellermann A, Aus dem Spring ES (2000) Ergebnisse und Komplikationen mit dem OATS-Instrumentarium. Arthroskopie 13:99–103
6. Buckwalter JA, Mankin HJ (1998) Articular cartilage repair and transplantation. Arthritis Rheum 41:1331–1342
7. Burkart AC, Schoettle P, Imhoff A (2001) Operative Therapiemöglichkeiten des Knorpelschadens. Unfallchirurg 104:798–807
8. Draenert K, Draenert Y (1988) A new procedure for bone biopsies and cartilage and bone transplantation. Sandorama III/IV:33–40
9. Garrett JC (1994) Fresh osteochondral allografts for treatment of articular defects in osteochondritis dissecans of the lateral femoral condyles in adults. Clin Orthop 303:33–37
10. Gautier E, Kolker D, Jakob RP (2002) Treatment of cartilage defects of the talus by autologous osteochondral grafts. J Bone Joint Surg-B 84:237–244
11. Goymann V (1999) Abrasionsarthroplastik. Orthopäde 28:11–18
12. Hangody L, Kish G, Karpati Z, Szerb I, Udvarhelyi I, Toth J, Dioszegi Z, Kendik Z (1997) Autogenous osteochondral graft technique for replacing knee cartilage defects. Orthop Intern 5:175–181
13. Hangody L, Kish G, Karpati Z, Szerb I, Udvarhelyi I (1997) Arthroscopic autogenous osteochondral mosaicplasty for the treatment of femoral condylar articular defects. Knee Surg Sports Traumatol Arthrosc 5:262–267
14. Hangody L, Kish G, Karpati Z, Udvarhelyi I, Szigeti I, Bely M (1998) Mosaicplasty for the treatment of articular cartilage defects: application in clinical practice. Orthopedics 21:751–756
15. Hangody L, Kish G, Modis L, Szerb I, Gaspar L, Dioszegi Z, Kendik Z (2001) Mosaicplasty for the treatment of osteochondritis dissecans of the talus: two to seven year results in 36 patients. Foot Ankle Int 22:552–558
16. Hangody L, Feczko P, Bartha L, Bodo G, Kish G (2001) Mosaicplasty for the treatment of articular defects of the knee and ankle. Clin Orthop 391 [Suppl]:328–336
17. Hochstein P, Schmickal T, Wentzensen A (2001) Autologes Resurfacing der Gelenkoberfläche. Trauma Berufskrankh 3:365–369
18. Imhoff AB, Öttl GM, Burkart A, Traub S (1999) Osteochondrale autologe Transplantation an verschiedenen Gelenken. Orthopäde 28:33–44
19. Imhoff AB, Burkart A, Öttl GM (1999) Der posteriore Kondylentransfer. Erste Erfahrungen mit einer Salvageoperation. Orthopäde 28:45–52
20. Jakob RP, Franz T, Gaultier E, Mainil-Varlet P (2002) Autologous osteochondral grafting in the knee: indication, results and reflections. Clin Orthop 401:170–184
21. Johnson LL (1991) Arthroscopic abrasion arthroplasty. In: McGinty JB (ed) Operative arthroscopy. Raven Press, New York, pp319–323
22. Laprell H, Petersen W (2001) Autologous osteochondral transplantation using the diamond bone-cutting system (DBCS): 6–12 years' follow-up of 35 patients with osteochondral defects at the knee joint. Arch Orthop Trauma Surg 121:248–253
23. Liebau C, Krämer R, Haak H, Baltzer A, Arnold J, Merk H, Krauspe R (2000) Technik der autologen Knorpel-Knochen-Transplantation. Arthroskopie 13:94–98
24. Mankin HJ (1982) The reponse of articular cartilage to mechanical injury. J Bone Joint Surg-A 64:460–466

25. Matsusue Y, Yamamuro T, Hma H (1993) Case report: Arthroscopic multiple osteochondral transplantation to the chondral defect in the knee associated with cruciate ligament disruption. Arthroscopy 9:318–321
26. Mueller B, Kohn D (1999) Indikation und Durchführung der Knorpel-Knochenanbohrung nach Pridie. Orthopäde 28:4–10
27. Outerbridge HK, Outerbridge AR, Outerbridge RE (1995) The use of lateral patellar autologous graft for the repair of a large osteochondral defect in the knee. J Bone Joint Surg-A 77:65–72
28. Peterson L, Minas T, Brittberg M, Nilsson A, Sjogren-Jansson E, Lindahl A (2000) Two- to 9-year outcome after autologous chondrocyte transplantation of the knee. Clin Orthop 374:212–235
29. Pridie KH (1959) A method of resurfacing osteoarthritic knee joints. J Bone Joint Surg-Br 41:618–619
30. Sammarco GJ, Makwana NK (2002) Treatment of talar osteochondral lesions using local osteochondral graft. Foot Ankle Int 23:693–698
31. Schoettle P, Oettl G, Agneskirchner J, Imhoff A (2001) Operative Therapie von osteochondralen Läsionen am Talus mit autologer Knorpel-Knochen-Transplantation. Orthopäde 30:53–58
32. Siebert CH, Miltner O, Schneider U, Wahner T, Koch S, Niedhart C (2001) Einheilungsverhalten von osteochondralen Transplantaten – Tierexperimentelle Untersuchungen an einem Schafmodell. Z Orthop 139:382–386
33. Simonian PT, Sussmann PS, Wickiewicz TL, Paletta GA, Warren RF (1998) Contact pressures at osteochondral donor sites at the knee. Am J Sports Med 26:491–494
34. Steadman JR, Rodkey WG, Briggs KK, Rodrigo JJ (1999) Die Technik der Mikrofrakturierung zur Behandlung von kompletten Knorpeldefekten im Kniegelenk. Orthopäde 28:26–32
35. Wagner H (1964) Operative Behandlung der Osteochondrosis dissecans des Kniegelenkes. Z Orthop 98:333–355
36. Wagner H (1972) Möglichkeiten und Erfahrungen mit der Knorpeltransplantation. Z Orthop 110:708–715
37. Wirth T, Rauch G, Schuler P, Griss P (1991) Das autologe Knorpel-Knochen-Transplantat zur Therapie der Osteochondrosis dissecans des Kniegelenkes. Z Orthop 129:80–84
38. Yamashita F, Sakakida K, Suzu F, Takai S (1985) The transplantation of an autogeneic osteochondral fragment for osteochondritis dissecans of the knee. Clin Orthop 201:43–50

Tissue Engineering

III

CHAPTER 8

Engineering Cartilage Structures* **8**

MICHAEL SITTINGER

The basic tissue engineering principle of musculoskeletal tissue repair is the delivery of functionally active cells within an appropriate carrier system to the damaged site, with a view to restore the original architecture and function of pathologically altered tissue. This approach comprises the interactive triad of responsive cells, a supportive matrix, and bioactive molecules promoting differentiation and regeneration. New developments in cell culturing techniques, delivery systems and materials, and regenerative concepts for the engineering of cartilage tissue are discussed.

After more than one decade of continuing research in tissue engineering, a growing number of cell-based therapies is emerging to achieve biological regeneration of damaged tissues or organs. The current technical approaches in cartilage tissue engineering are typically based on artificial tissue constructs of autologous cells and biomaterials that function as a cell-embedding component and/or as a scaffold for the formation of three-dimensional tissues (Fig. 8.1).

Experimental approaches to engineer skeletal tissue transplants vary considerably between the different intended clinical indications. *In vitro* formation of external ear cartilage demands particular attention to tissue pre-shaping and *in vivo* shape stabilization [5]. Joint cartilage regeneration involves special techniques to handle and anchor cells and tissues in the joint defect. So far, successful preliminary clinical studies have shown that *in vitro* engineering and transplantation of autologous cartilage tissues is possible.

However, new strategies for the regeneration of severely degenerated cartilage surfaces in osteoarthritis and in chronic inflammatory joint diseases are still in an experimental state. These next-generation tissue engineering therapies will be increasingly based on the regenerative potential of stem cells and morphogenic growth factors which will be used to induce healing *in vivo*.

Culturing Techniques and Cells

Although frequently used in tissue engineering approaches, conventional monolayer cultures of autologous cells have their limitations in generating highly differentiated

---

* Reprinted with permission from Sittinger M (2003) Engineering cartilage structures. In: Sandell L (ed) Tissue engineering. American Academy of Orthopaedic Surgeons, Rosemont. In press.

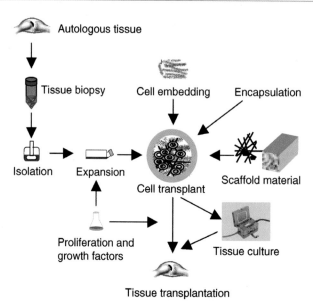

Autologous tissue

Tissue biopsy   Cell embedding   Encapsulation

Isolation   Expansion

Cell transplant   Scaffold material

Proliferation and growth factors

Tissue culture

Tissue transplantation

Fig. 8.1.
General procedure for autologous tissue replacement. The isolation and selection of autologous cells from tissue biopsies is followed by *ex vivo* expansion. Expanded cells are embedded within a suitable biomatrix. Cell-matrix composites are either cultured in perfusion chambers or directly implanted into a lesion.

structures. The reasons for this are as follows: metabolic conditions within the culture medium are unstable and not comparable to the *in vivo* situation; no extracellular matrix (ECM) is formed and consequently important cell-cell and cell-ECM interactions can not take place; mesenchymal cells tend to de-differentiate in monolayer cultures (e.g. chondrocytes transform into fibroblasts) [1, 10].

To optimize the medium composition, but also to approach the specific challenges related to the culturing of organoid arrangements, such as high nutrient consumption (due to high densities) and presence of supportive delivery materials, artificial tissue constructs are cultured in bioreactors. Perfusion of these reactors permits the stabilization of culture medium components, the maintenance of secreted autocrine factors (such as morphogenic signals) at a desired level, and the avoidance of an overshoot in synthesized paracrine factors, thereby mimicking the *in vivo* situation [17]. Additional progress might be achieved by the use of gradient chambers. By these means, a concentration gradient of differentiating morphogenic factors could be established across the artificial tissues which would be similar to the situation pertaining during embryonic development.

To support ECM formation and normal cell-cell interactions, three-dimensional cell culturing systems have proved to be successful [12, 14]. Obviously, such systems (e.g. scaffolds or gels) mimic the *in vivo* situation quite well, because grown in these settings, cells do not de-differentiate or even re-differentiate to their original phenotype [1]. New developments in this area will be discussed below.

Today, most tissue repair approaches involving autologous cells take the use of biopsies from healthy sites of the tissue in question. Although the use of these differentiated cells has proved to be successful in many approaches, it also involves several problems: the availability of cells might be restricted, the site of sampling becomes severely damaged and with respect to their functional termination not all cells types are able to proliferate *in vitro*. In view of these problems, research is increasingly focusing on tissue regeneration involving precursor or multipotent stem cells. Mesenchymal stem cells from the bone marrow appear to be good candidates for tissue repair therapies: they are easy to obtain, are of autologous origin, have the capacity for unlimited but controlled expansion and have the potential to differentiate into various mesenchymal tissues depending on the microenvironment. Indeed, under defined culture conditions, uncommitted mesenchymal progenitor cells from bone marrow have been shown to differentiate into chondrocytes [6].

Delivery Materials

In joint cartilage replacement, pressure resistance and fixation of the transplant onto the bone is more important and difficult than in plastic surgery. In theory, the artificially grown cartilage layers could be attached directly to the defective joint surface using fibrin glue, resorbable sutures, pins or staples. Other promising approaches focus on osteochondral replacements, such as artificial cartilage attached directly on porous calcium carbonate for subchondral bone repair [8].

Until recently, focal articular cartilage defects have been treated mainly by injecting suspensions of cartilage cells into a lesion that is covered by a small periosteal flap [2]. Today, the deployment of fully developed or pre-shaped cartilage transplants is in progress. The formation of such three-dimensional tissues is achieved using different scaffold structures. Especially during the initial post-transplantation phase, these scaffolds provide mechanical stability; they also ensure a homogeneous and efficient distribution of the cells within their confines and thus within the cartilage lesion to be repaired.

The materials used for these matrices have to be biocompatible, i.e., they should neither provoke an immunological rejection reaction nor influence the normal metabolic activities of cells. The intrinsic structure of the matrix should allow the homogeneous distribution of a sufficient number of cells within its structure and support a close contact between newly synthesized ECM molecules and cells – pre-requisites for the spatial maturation of the tissue. Furthermore, the matrix should exhibit a homogeneous structure and be flexible, but still sufficiently stable to permit the firm fixation or arthroscopic implantation of cultured cartilage material. After prolonged cultivation, the tissue becomes stabilized by the newly formed ECM and the supportive matrix is no longer required. Therefore, a biodegradable scaffold material is recommended, which can be resorbed after a certain period of time without interfering with the metabolic activity of the maturing tissue [15].

Fibers

Polymer fiber constructs consisting of poly(α-hydroxyesters) meet the aforementioned requirements most closely. These resorbable fibers can form e.g. a three-dimensional fleece that is flexible and robust and that can be shaped to meet anatomical requirements. Having a low material-to-volume ratio, these fiber structures effectively promote the three-dimensional growth of cells.

When loading the fleeces with cells, the latter tend to sink out of the fiber structure. To avoid this, chondrocytes can either be directly attached to the fibers, using e.g. adhesion factors, or be embedded in gel-like substances [15], such as agarose, fibrin or hyaluronic acid, which permit a homogeneous distribution of cells within the carrier. Gel-like substances permit an increase in the average distance between fibers, which further reduces the total amount of polymer per tissue volume. In this combination, the fibers serve as a scaffold for the tissue, while the gels are responsible for the three-dimensional distribution of the cells (Fig. 8.2). An alternative approach which aims to accumulate cells and especially matrix molecules within the fiber structure involves encapsulating the whole structure in a semi-permeable membrane [16].

Collagen matrices exhibit a high cell-binding capacity. However, collagen is known to rapidly loose its mechanical stability when maintained in culture media, and when using e.g. collagen type I for production, the characteristics of the matrices formed are not always consistent. Furthermore, weak interconnections between cavities, as well as low porosity, tend to impede the optimal three-dimensional distribution of cells. Implantation of collagen into articular cartilage lesions without the addition of cells leads to wound closure. However, the newly formed tissue is rather low in proteoglycans, which are decisive for the elasticity of the transplant [18].

Hydrogels

In contrast to polymer fibers, gels do not provide the stability that is required for the *in vitro* formation of cartilage transplants. However, the direct injection of cell-carrying gels into a lesion may be used to treat smaller defects [13]. Hydrogels mimic several distinct structural and physico-chemical characteristics of the ECM, which is likewise a gel, consisting of hyaluronic acid, proteoglycans and supportive collagen fibers.

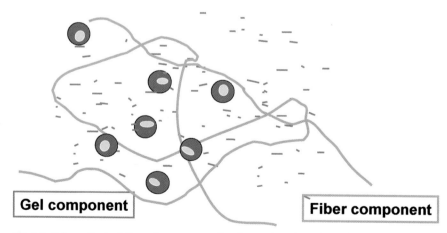

Gel component   **Fiber component**

Fig. 8.2. Schematic depiction of a construct for the engineering of cartilage tissue based on fibers and an embedding substance. The embedding substance ensures the three-dimensional immobilization and uniform distribution of cells within the fibrous meshwork.

Agarose gels are frequently used for chondrogenesis research. However they are rarely used for the generation of transplants in that immunological aspects of the agarose and its degradation products have to be clarified. Within agarose gels, the distance between cells is relatively large. While this gives ECM components sufficient space to aggregate [23], large molecules, such as aggrecan, remain in the peri-cellular domain, impeding the formation of a connecting intercellular matrix [22].

Fibrin gels are commonly used in surgical medicine and they provide the biocompatibility required. Since the mechanical stability of fibrin gels is rather limited, a combination of these gels with more stable components is recommended. Promising results have been achieved using a chondrocyte-carrying fibrin gel that was mechanically stabilized with a resorbable polymer fleece (Fig. 8.3). This combination facilitated optimal handling during surgery, exhibited satisfactory mechanical stability and permitted a homogeneous three-dimensional distribution of cells within the transplant [11].

Alginate is an immobilization matrix, within which chondrocytes are able to generate an ECM and maintain their phenotype *in vitro*. The subcutaneous implantation of alginate beads covered with chondrocytes has yielded tissue (30% to 40% cartilage) that became wrapped by a fibrous tissue capsule within 6 weeks after implantation [3]. When alginate beads are combined with hyaluromic acid or fibrin gels, the number of cells that can be trapped within the beads increases substantially [9]. However, the deployment of alginate as an implant carrier is still under discussion, owing to doubts about the purity of the material and its immunological behavior.

Hyaluromic acid (HA) chains form networks which represent useful carrier matrices [19]. Depending on the type of linking reaction, either fibers or gels can be generated. Low levels of linkage are associated with advanced water uptake into the gels. Although this weakens the mechanical stability of a hyaluromic acid matrix, it increases its biodegradability and has a positive impact on the generation of a physiologically relevant tissue pressure within the transplant.

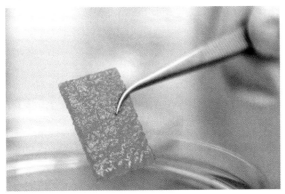

Fig. 8.3. *In vitro* engineered cartilage construct for the treatment of joint defects. Such an engineered construct has been applied arthroscopically to cartilage lesions.
This illustration is printed with kind permission by the Arthroscopy: Erggelet C, Sittinger M, Lahm A,: The arthroscopic implantation of autologous chondrocytes for the treatment of full-thickness cartilage defects of the knee joint. Arthroscopy, 2003 Jan; 19(1):108–110, WB Sounders Company an Elsevier Scientist Company; © 2003 The Arthroscopy Association of North America)

Evolution of Regenerative Concepts

Despite the promising approaches described above, the treatment of more extensive joint lesions is still problematic. In particular, the restricted potential of cultured chondrocytes to proliferate and subsequently differentiate impedes the generation of larger portions of replacement tissue with a sufficient stability and adequate structure. Moreover, musculoskeletal structures such as the joint comprise a morphological and functional unit, and pathological changes are never restricted to a single tissue.

Novel strategies aim to circumvent these shortcomings by focusing on chondro- and e.g. bone-inductive stimuli to regenerate cartilage and other joint tissues in a concerted manner *in vivo*. Preliminary investigations have been performed using bone morphogenic protein-2 (BMP-2) or transforming growth factor-(β)-1. Injection of these factors into the joint induced the formation of type II collagen and the synthesis of proteoglycans by chondrocytes and therefore cartilage growth and maturation [21]. In another approach, osteochondral defects of rabbit knees were treated with collagen sponges coated with human BMP-2. Histological staining for type II collagen and proteoglycans revealed the formation of normal cartilage tissue after 24 weeks *in vivo* [20]. Thus, BMP-2 may be a promising candidate for the engineering of cartilage tissue in joint defects. In the case of destructive joint diseases such as osteoarthritis and rheumatoid arthritis, BMP-7 has successfully promoted the differentiation and stabilization of cartilage tissue [7]. It is likely that inductive regenerative treatments will involve a sequential cascade of more than one factor to trigger first cell migration and proliferation and subsequently the differentiation and maturation of induced regenerating tissues. The combination of such approaches with the cell/scaffold composites described above will be an important step forward in cartilage tissue engineering.

Future Directions

The following aspects are expected to strongly influence the future directions of joint cartilage regeneration.

Stem Cells

Future research and development in cartilage regeneration will have to define the favorite options of cell source. It is generally assumed that stem cells have great potential in tissue engineering. However, it is still uncertain if stem or precursor cells derived from different tissues will actually result in better treatment results or more convenient concepts in cartilage repair.

Allogenic Cell Sources

Cell treatments based on other than autologous cells would significantly facilitate production and logistics of tissue engineering products. However, considering a rather perfect human immune system, a long-term survival of any allogenic cells will be very difficult to achieve even when transplanted cells are modified to reduce cellular immune responses.

In Vivo Regeneration

Therapies based on *in situ* tissue engineering will have tremendous potential, as it would then be possible to avoid costly cell culture procedures for each individual patient. One or a whole cascade of growth, differentiation and chemotactic factors in suitable delivery systems would have to replace the regenerative inductive signals normally provided by the transplanted cells in conventional tissue engineering approaches.

References

1. Benya PD, Shaffer JD (1982) Dedifferentiated chondrocytes re-express the differentiated collagen phenotype when cultured in agarose gels. Cell 30:215–224
2. Brittberg M, Lindahl A, Nilsson A, Ohlsson C, Isaksson O, Peterson L (1994) Treatment of deep cartilage defects in the knee with autologous chondrocyte transplantation. N Engl J Med 331:889–895
3. Cao Y, Rodriguez A, Vacanti M, Ibarra C, Arevalo C, Vacanti CA (1998) Comparative study of use of poly(glycolic acid), calcium alginate and pluronics in the engineering of autologous porcine cartilage. J Biomater Sci Polym Ed 9:475–487
4. Erggelet C, Sittinger M, Lahm A (2003) The arthroscopic implantation of autologous chondrocytes for the treatment of full-thickness cartilage defects of the knee joint. Arthroscopy 19:108–110
5. Haisch A, Klaring S, Groger A, Gebert C, Sittinger M (2002) A tissue-engineering model for the manufacture of auricular-shaped cartilage implant. Eur Arch Otorhinolaryngol 259:316–312
6. Kadiyala S, Young RG, Thiede MA, Bruder SP (1997) Culture expanded canine mesenchymal stem cells possess osteochondrogenic potential in vivo and in vitro. Cell Transplant 6:125–134
7. Kaps C, Bramlage C, Smolian H et al. (2002) Bone morphogenetic proteins promote cartilage differentiation and protect engineered artificial cartilage from fibroblast invasion and destruction. Arthritis Rheum 46:149–162
8. Kreklau B, Sittinger M, Mensing MB et al. (1999) Tissue engineering of biphasic joint cartilage transplants. Biomaterials 20:1743–1749
9. Lindenhayn K, Perka C, Spitzer R, Heilmann H, Pommerening K, Mennicke J, Sittinger M (1998) Retention of hyaluronic acid in alginate beads: Aspects for in vitro cartilage engineering. Biomed Mater Res 44:149–155
10. Minuth WW, Sittinger M, Kloth S (1998) Tissue engineering – generation of differential artificial tissues for biomedical applications. Cell Tiss Res 291:1–11
11. Perka C, Sittinger M, Schultz O, Spitzer RS, Schlenzka D, Burmester GR (2000) Tissue engineered cartilage repair using cryopreserved and noncryopreserved chondrocytes. Clin Orthop 378:245–254
12. Risbud MV, Sittinger M (2002) Tissue engineering: advances in in vitro cartilage generation. Trends Biotechnol 20:351–356
13. Risbud M, Ringe J, Bhonde R, Sittinger M (2001) In vitro expression of cartilage-specific markers by chondrocytes on a biocompatible hydrogel: implications for engineering cartilage tissue. Cell Transplant 10:775–763
14. Schultz O, Sittinger M, Haeupl T, Burmester GR (2000) Emerging strategies of bone and joint repair. Arthritis Res 2:433–436

15. Sittinger M, Bujia J, Rotter N, Reitzel D, Minuth WW, Burmester GR (1996) Tissue engineering and autologous transplant formation: practical approaches with resorbable biomaterials and new cell culture techniques. Biomaterials 17:237–242
16. Sittinger M, Lukanoff B, Burmester GR, Dautzenberg H (1996) Encapsulation of artificial tissues in polyelectrolyte complexes: Preliminary studies. Biomaterials 17:1049–1051
17. Sittinger M, Schultz O, Keyszer G, Minuth WW, Burmester GR (1997) Artificial tissues in perfusion culture. Int J Artif Org 20:57–62
18. Speer DP, Chvapil M, Volz RG, Holmes MD (1991) Enhancement of healing in osteochondral defects by collagen sponge implants. Clin Orthop 144:326–335
19. Tomihata K, Ikada Y (1997) Preparation of cross-linked hyaluronic acid films of low water content. Biomaterials 18:189–195
20. van Beuningen HM, Glansbeek HL, Kraan van der PM, Berg van den WB (1998) Differential effects of local application of BMP-2 or TGF-(beta)1 on both articular cartilage compositions and osteophyte formation. Ostheoarthritis Cartilage 6:306–317
21. van Beuningen HM, Glansbeek HL, Kraan van der PM, Berg van den WB (2000) Osteoarthritis-like changes in the murine knee joint resulting from intra-articular transforming growth factor-(beta) injection. Ostheoarthritis Cartilage 8:25–33
22. Verbruggen G, Veys EM, Wieme N, Malfait AM, Gijselbrecht L, Nimmegrees J, Almquist KF, Broddelez C (1990) The synthesis and immobilization of cartilage-specific proteoglycan by human chondrocytes in different concentrations of agarose. Clin Exp Rheumatol 8:371–378
23. von Schroeder HP, Kwan M, Amiel D, Coutts RD (1991) The use of polylactic acid matrix and periostal grafts for the reconstruction of rabbit knee articular defects. J Biomed Mater Res 25:329–339

Biomaterials

Homogeneously Cross-Linked Scaffolds Based on Clinical-Grade Alginate for Transplantation and Tissue Engineering*

9

ULRICH ZIMMERMANN, ULRICH LEINFELDER, MARKUS HILLGÄRTNER, BERTRAM MANZ, HEIKO ZIMMERMANN, FRANK BRUNNENMEIER, MIKE WEBER, JULIO A. VÁSQUEZ, FRANK VOLKE and CHRISTIAN HENDRICH

Introduction

Transplantation of therapeutic allogenic tissues or genetically manipulated cells without immunosuppression is a promising strategy for the long-term treatment of various hormone deficiencies and neuro-degenerative diseases in human [9, 8, 18]. To achieve this promise, host reactions against the transplants must be prevented by encapsulation in a microcapsule. A major problem of encapsulation is the precise adjustment of the numerous matrix- and host-related parameters to the need of immunoisolation, while not impeding simultaneously the inward transport of nutrients and oxygen and the release of the generated therapeutic factors from the microcapsule core. Numerous animal studies and recent pilot clinical trials have shown the feasibility of alginate-based microcapsules for long-term immunoisolated transplantation [5, 18]. Alginate also has many potential advantages as a tissue engineering matrix [2, 14]. The primary challenge in the field of regenerative medicine is to promote formation of missing or non-functioning tissue by transplantation of specialized autologous cells. Repair of articular cartilage lesions by mesenchymal stem cells or chrondrocytes is one of the key applications. In this case, the alginate matrix serves as a three-dimensional scaffold for promotion of re-differentiation and formation of hyaline cartilage by *in vitro* expanded and de-differentiated cells.

Designing of an alginate matrix for immunoisolated transplantation and tissue engineering must meet a set of stringent requirements for alginate production, purity level and characterization as well as for microcapsule manufacture. Formulation of an alginate matrix must be performed in accordance with GMP/ISO 9000 and the guidelines for safety criteria, which are given by the American Society for Testing and Materials (ASTM; quoted in [3]).

* We are very grateful to M. Behringer, P. Geßner and A. Steinbach for skillful technical assistance. This work was supported by grants from the Landesgewerbeanstalt (High-Tech-Offensive des Freistaates Bayern), the Deutsche Forschungsgemeinschaft (DFG, Zi 99/16–1) and the BMBF (VDI 16SV1329) given to U. Z., by grants from FONDECYT 1000044 to J.A.V., by grants from the Deutsche Forschungsgemeinschaft (He 2460/4–1) to C. H., by a grant from BMBF (VDI 16SV1366/0) to H. Z., and by grants from IBMT to F. V.

This article focuses on the exploitation of parameters that determine the success of alginate-based transplants. Solutions are presented for designing microcapsules that may obtain regulatory approval for clinical applications in the near future.

Requirements for Producing Clinical-Grade Alginates

Alginates are natural anionic polymers isolated from marine brown algae. The hydrogels are a family of non-branched binary copolymers of 1- to 4-glycosidically-linked β-D-mannuronic acid (M) and α-L-glucoronic acid (G) residues. The monomers are sequenced in homopolymeric G-G-G and M-M-M blocks interspaced with blocks of alternating sequence (M-G-M). Alginates extracted from different algal material can vary both in monomer composition and block arrangement, and this has direct influence on the physico-chemical properties of the (cross-linked) hydrogel (e.g. viscosity, gel-forming, swelling properties, mechanical strength etc.) [7]. Alginates, which exhibit an M:G ratio of 70:30 yield best transplantation results [16, 18–20]. Sources of this material are peeled stipes of *Laminaria pallida* and particularly of *Lessonia nigrescens*, both harvested from the sea [10].

The starting algal material is naturally contaminated by mitogenic and cytotoxic compounds (including heavy metal ions) [15, 19]. Critically there are also bacterial- and animal-originating impurities, varying greatly with the pollution of the sea, as well as with the weather and surf conditions at the collection site. Part of these impurities are removed during the extraction process, but spores of gram-negative and particularly of gram-positive bacteria together with related compounds will be found in the final alginate product. Some of these contaminants also induce de-polymerization of the polymer chains, thus leading to alginates of low viscosity (i.e. low molecular mass) which are immunoreactive. This requires that these contaminants are eliminated before the manufacturing process. Thus, the act of harvesting and subsequent drying process of the algal material is extremely crucial and must obligatorily include appropriate steps for bacterial removal.

Large scale manufacture of clinical-grade quality alginate, using the described algal material as the input source, can be achieved by subjecting the material to EDTA extraction, filtration and three consecutive ethanol precipitation steps [20]. The viscosity of the final product (and in turn of the average molecular mass) is extremely high compared to the viscosity of commercial (contaminated) alginates. Depending on the species the viscosity of a 0.1% (w/v in distilled water) alginate solution can assume values around 30 mPa s (versus 1 to 5 mPa s measured for a 0.1% [w/v in distilled water] solution of commercial alginate).

Quality Assessment

Ultra-high viscosity (UHV) alginate is extremely biocompatible for both the host and the cells it encloses, provided that bacteria-free algal material is used for extraction. Current routine analytical assays for testing the purity of alginates comprise measurements of endotoxin, protein and phenolic-like compounds by using the limulus-lysate assay, the Bradford test, fluorescence- and NMR-spectroscopy, respectively. Measurements of alginates extracted from algal material that is not bacteria-free show, however, that these analytical assays are not sufficient to exclude immunological reactions upon transplantation of alginate microcapsules underneath the kidney capsule of spontaneously diabetic BB rats. This strain is the most stringent small animal model to date, presumably because of its elevated macrophage activity. Data obtained in this model can be easily extrapolated to the clinical situation in human. As shown in Fig. 9.1 the immunological response to Ba^{2+}-cross-linked alginate microcapsules

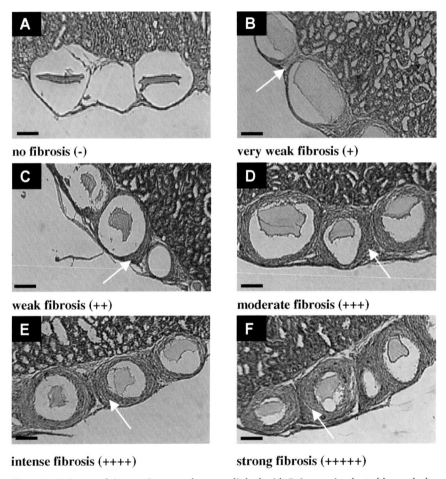

Fig. 9.1A–F. Empty alginate microcapsules cross-linked with Ba^{2+} were implanted beneath the kidney capsules of spontaneously diabetic BB rats. To manufacture the microcapsules, ultra-high viscosity alginates were used that were extracted from fresh stipes of *Laminaria pallida* and *Lessonia nigrescens*, and harvested from the sea or collected at the beach. Note that implants shown in **F** were made from commercial alginate. After 3 weeks the implants were retrieved and processed for histological analysis (HE staining). The different degrees of fibrosis (*arrows*) evoked by the various alginate samples were assigned with "+" signs ranging from "–" for no fibrosis (**A**) to five "+" for strong fibrosis (**F**). Bar = 150 µm (for more details, see [10]).

could range from no fibrotic reactions (Fig. 9.1A; alginate extracted from bacteria-free *L. nigrescens algae*) to strong fibrotic overgrowth (Fig. 9.1F; commercial alginate). Alginates extracted from bacteria-containing stipes of *Laminaria pallida* and *Lessonia nigrescens* provoked very varying responses ranging from very weak (+) over weak (++) and moderate (+++) up to intense (++++) fibrotic reactions (Fig. 9.1B–E). When stipes harvested from the sea were used as an input source the immuno-reactivity was on average much less than that observed for alginates extracted from fresh stipes collected at the beach (see also Table 9.1). Foreign body reactions denoted by the sign (+) apparently do not prevent nutrient, oxygen and factor transfer between the core of the microcapsule and the environment, and are thus acceptable for transplantation. Fibrotic reactions, denoted by the sign (++) are clearly not satisfactory, but can still be classified under some circumstances as relatively biocompatible provided that optimal nutrient supply is guaranteed by vascularization of the microcapsules. In contrast, alginate displaying immunoreactivity denoted by three or more plus signs (+++), is certainly inappropriate for tissue engineering and immunoisolated transplantation. For a quantitative characterization of the varying results of the rodent studies a fibrotic index was introduced according to Leinfelder et al. [10]. To this end, the value "0" was assigned for no fibrosis (–), and accordingly values "1" to "5" for very weak (+) up to strong fibrosis (+++++). The mean ± standard deviation of the fibrotic values was taken as an estimate for the average frequency of fibrosis induced by a certain alginate (Table 9.1).

The immunoreactivity pattern of alginates extracted from untreated and bacteria-free stipes is also seen in an apoptosis assay recently developed in our laboratory [10]. The assay is based on the shift of the emitted fluorescence of the fluorescence cyanine

Table 9.1. Fibrotic versus apoptotic and mitogenic indices

	Commercial alginate	Ultra-high viscosity alginates			
Species	Not specified	L. pallida stipes		L. nigrescens stipes	
Collection site	Not specified	Sea	Beach	Sea	Sea[2]
Apoptotic index	0.77 ± 0.03 (72)	1.13 ± 0.05 (27)	1.55 ± 0.06 (38)	1.09 ± 0.04 (43)	1.06 ± 0.04 (26)
Mitogenic index	2.03 ± 0.14 (13)	0.56 ± 0.08 (12)	0.56 ± 0.04 (29)	0.67 ± 0.11 (8)	0.66 ± 0.03 (21)
Fibrotic index	4.80 ± 0.13 (10)	2.50 ± 0.23 (18)	3.66 ± 0.23 (12)	1.45 ± 0.16 (11)	0.75 ± 0.25 (4)

[a] Data are given as mean ± standard deviation; number of measurements are given in brackets. Note that in the absence of apoptotic and mitogenic impurities the corresponding indices are 1.00. With increasing concentrations of apoptotic or mitogenic impurities the indices assume increasingly higher values than 1.00. Apoptotic indices lower than 1.00 are measured when the alginate contains mitogenic contaminants, as is the case of commercial alginate. Mitogenic indices lower than 1.00 are expected when the alginates have suppressed the mitogenity of the lipopolysaccharides. For further details, see text and [10].

[b] Bacteria were removed before the stipes were extracted.

dye JC-1 from red to green upon apoptosis, which can be measured *via* flow cytometry [1, 13]. The percentage ratio of green fluorescent cells in alginate-treated cells to green fluorescent cells in untreated cells is the so-called apoptotic index and can be taken as a measure for apoptosis-inducing contaminants in the alginate (see Table 9.1). The assay offers very sensitive detection of apoptosis-inducing impurities in alginates, when human Jurkat T-cell leukemia cells after more than 20 passages are used. Mitogenic impurities can interfere with this assay, thus leading to wrong interpretations. Therefore, these contaminants must be determined separately by using the modified "mixed-lymphocyte" test. As shown by Zimmermann et al. [17] the proliferation of the lymphocytes in the presence of mitogenic impurities can greatly be enhanced when the cells are simultaneously co-stimulated by bacterial lipopolysaccharides. Further improvement of reproducibility and sensitivity can be achieved if the number and size of the proliferating cells are determined electronically [20]. The area beneath the size distribution of the proliferating cells in relation to the area of the size distribution of the control cells stimulated only with lipopolysaccharide is the so-called mitogenic index and is an estimate for the concentration of mitogenic impurities in the alginate (see Table 9.1).

Inspection of Table 9.1 shows that differences in BB-rat-immunoreactivity of alginates extracted from beach and sea, as well as of alginates extracted from bacteria-free stipes and bacteria-containing stipes could clearly be resolved by using the apoptotic assay. However, as demonstrated for commercial alginates the apoptotic index can not be used as a measure for the purity of alginates when the mitogenic index is ≥1. Interestingly, the mitogenic index of the UHV-alginates is <1, indicating that alginate suppressed the mitogenic activity of lipopolysaccharides.

Design of Microcapsules

Ca^{2+} and Ba^{2+} ions are usually used for cross-linking of the carboxyl groups of the polymeric alginate chains. Ca^{2+} cross-linked microcapsules are dissolved by citrate, phosphate, lactate, and other chelators because of the relatively low affinity constant of these divalent ions to alginate. Thus, gelling with Ca^{2+} is not recommended for long-term immunoisolated transplantation, but can be advantageous when autologous cells are transplanted because the alginate matrix serves only as a temporary scaffold in this case. The *in vitro* and *in vivo* long-term integrity of the microcapsules is greatly improved when Ba^{2+} is used [4]. However, these capsules still show a high tendency to take up large amounts of water, which causes them to swell in saline solutions, leading ultimately to disintegration and under *in vivo* conditions to graft failure (6, 11, 18–20). Swelling can be greatly reduced if perfluorocarbons, 10% fetal calf serum (FCS) or 1% human serum albumin (HSA) are added to the alginate solution, before cross-linking. Perfluorocarbons and HSA have the advantage that medical approval is granted. Perfluorocarbons are additionally beneficial because they improve the oxygen transfer in the alginate matrix and allow long-term visualization of the transplants under non-invasive conditions by using ^{19}F-NMR [18, 19]. The removal of excessive Ba^{2+} ions in the alginate matrix is of equal importance for microcapsule stability, as is the incorporation of swelling-suppressing agents. This can be achieved by washing the microcapsules at least 3 times with isotonic NaCl solution followed by sodium sulfate treatment, resulting in the formation of insoluble tiny $BaSO_4$ crystals.

Swelling and stability of the alginate matrix are also closely tied with the cross-linking process. Usually, the (cell- and additives-containing) alginate solution is forced through a syringe or through the nozzle of a two- or three-channel coaxial air-jet microcapsule generator [9, 19]. The droplets fall into a solution containing 20 mM $BaCl_2$, appropriate amounts of NaCl and buffer substances. However, when gelling is only performed from the external side, the core of the microcapsules remains uncross-linked because of great diffusion restrictions in the outermost cross-linked layer. The incomplete cross-linking of the alginate matrix can be demonstrated by confocal laser scanning microscopy (CLSM), the tiny $BaSO_4$ crystals. To this end, the microcapsules made of alginate extracted from *Lessonia nigrescens* stipes were washed only once before sulfate treatment, in order to avoid complete removal of the excessive Ba^{2+}. A typical optical section of a CLSM image of a microcapsule performed by the conventional cross-linking method is shown in Fig. 9.2A. Innumerable crystals can be seen at the periphery, but only a few, if any, within the core of the microcapsule.

It is evident that uniform cross-linking throughout the microcapsule requires approaches that allow a simultaneous internal gelling of the alginate. A possible way is to mix the alginate solution with caged Ba^{2+} before droplet formation. Caged ions are not reactive, but free reactive ions can easily be released by UV-irradiation once the droplets come in contact with the $BaCl_2$ solution [18, 19]. The drawback of this method is that the released organic cage compounds will not receive medical approval. Mixing the alginate solution with $BaCO_3$ and subsequently liberating the Ba^{2+} ions by the lower pH of the bath solution is also not suitable for medical applications. Due to the high affinity constant of Ba^{2+} to alginate the cross-linking process starts before droplet formation, leading to irregularly shaped microcapsules (which are inappropriate both for immunoisolated transplantation and tissue engineering). Other approaches reported in the literature also have decisive drawbacks (quoted in [21]).

The problems of the lack of internal gelling have recently been overcome by the so-called crystal gun method [21]. With this technique, simultaneous internal and external cross-linking of the alginate polymeric chains is achieved by injection of $BaCl_2$ crystals into the fluid alginate droplets before they come in contact with the bath solution containing 20 mM $BaCl_2$. This produces guarantees a homogeneous distribution of Ba^{2+} throughout the microcapsules, as shown by the optical CLSM section through a cross-linked microcapsule (see Fig. 9.2B) as opposed to the microcapsule cross-linked without using the crystal gun (see Fig. 9.2A). The improved cross-linking of the alginate droplets achieved by using the crystal gun method is also demonstrated by T_1-weighted NMR micro-imaging of microcapsules made of alginate extracted from *Lessonia nigrescens* stipes and cross-linked with Cu^{2+}. This divalent ion has the same affinity constant for alginate as Ba^{2+}, but has the great advantage over Ba^{2+} that it reduces the T_1-relaxation time of its molecular surrounding. The surfaces reconstructed from three-dimensional images of 11-day old microcapsules made by using the conventional cross-linking technique and the crystal gun method are given in Figs. 9.2C and D, respectively. It is clear that injection of $CuSO_4$ crystals into the alginate droplets leads to a very uniform bulk cross-linking of the alginate, resulting in solid microcapsules with clearly separated shapes (Fig. 9.2D). In

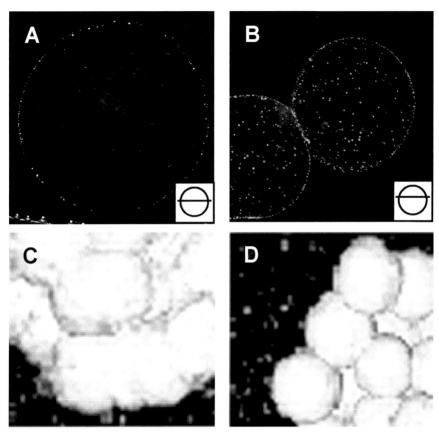

Fig. 9.2A–D. Confocal laser scanning microscopy images (**A,B**) and reconstructed surface images obtained from three-dimensional NMR images (**C,D**) of alginate microcapsules (about 800 μm in diameter). The microcapsules were made of 0.8% alginate extracted from *Lessonia nigrescens* and cross-linked by using the conventional cross-linking method (*left side* of the panel) and the crystal gun method (*right side* of the panel). The microcapsules in **A,B** were cross-linked with Ba^{2+}, stabilized with protein and washed once with NaCl solution before excess Ba^{2+} was precipitated by sulfate treatment. The scans were performed in the reflection mode of an air-cooled argon laser at 488 nm line, thus visualizing the $BaSO_4$ clusters. The insets on the right lower side of both images give the approximate focal plane. The microcapsules in **C,D** were cross-linked with Cu^{2+} (because of its effect on the T1-relaxation time of NMR micro-imaging). Before use, the microcapsules were stored in 0.9% NaCl solution for 11 days. The images were acquired at a magnetic field strength of 9.7 Tesla using a T1-weighted 3D spin-echo sequence (for more details, see [21]).

contrast, microcapsules made conventionally exhibit strong disintegration as indicated by flowing into one another (Fig. 9.2C). Internal gelling also results in very smooth surfaces provided that excessive Ba^{2+} is removed. This can be demonstrated by atomic force microscopy images (AFM) of the microcapsule surfaces. As shown in Fig. 9.3A microcapsules stored for 2 days in the Ba^{2+} cross-linking solution show cor-

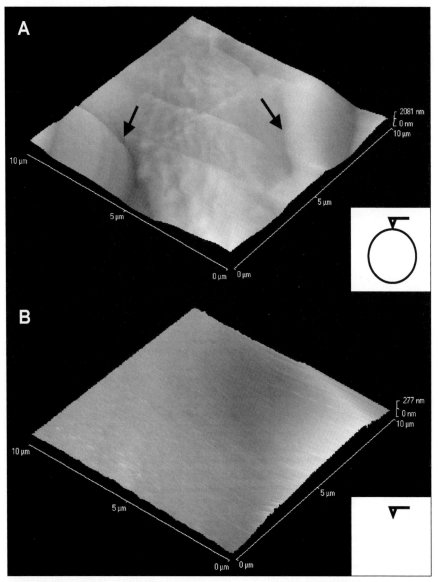

Fig. 9.3A,B. Atomic force microscope surface images of two empty Ba^{2+} alginate microcapsules made of 0.8% alginate, extracted from *Lessonia nigrescens,* stabilized with 10% FCS and produced using the crystal gun method. The capsule in **A** was stored in the $BaCl_2$ solution for 2 days before the scan was performed. The scan range is 10×10 μm^2 and the height scale is 2081 nm. The area roughness is 223.5 nm. The surface reveals corrugations and crevices (*arrows*). To emphasize these features the picture is presented in the so-called shadow mode. The capsule in **B** was washed 3 times with NaCl solution, treated with sulfate and kept in NaCl solution for 6 days. In contrast to **A** the surface is quite homogenous. The maximum height is 277 nm, the scan range is 10×10 μm^2. The area roughness value is 29.3 nm. Both images were acquired in the non-contact mode under liquid environment. The scans were performed at the top of the alginate capsules (see insets).

rugations and crevices whereas the surface of washed and sulfate-treated microcapsules is nearly homogeneous (Fig. 9.3B). Smooth surfaces of transplants are important, because it is well known that the immunological response of the host is not only determined by the chemical reactivity of the biomaterial, but also by the topography of the surface. While purified alginates can not serve as a substrate for cell attachment [19], tiny surface imperfections present suitable targets for the attachment and subsequent spreading, migration, and growth of anchorage dependent cells. Migrating cells, however, regularly release material traces [16, 17]. These can react with the guluronic and mannuronic acids under formation of immunogenic advanced glycation end products (quoted in [19]). Fibrotic reactions or even microcapsule disintegration are also induced by further attachment of macrophages and other anchorage-dependent cells.

Encapsulation of rat Langerhans' islets, of human monoclonal antibody secreting hybridoma cells, and of murine BMP-transfected mesenchymal stem cells has given clear-cut evidence (see chapter 2) [11, 21] that injection of $BaCl_2$ crystals into the microcapsules has no compromising effect on cell viability and function. These investigations have also shown [11] that the network of the cross-linked polymeric chains of the alginate is very tight. Slightly lower alginate concentrations must be used in order to obtain optimum nutrient and oxygen transfer, as well as unimpeded release of the therapeutic factors from the microcapsule core. Further, lowering of the alginate concentration leads to cross-linked matrices, which have less stability. Such cross-linked alginates are promising scaffolds for tissue engineering, e.g. for repair of cartilage lesions (see chapter 2).

Conclusion

The large-scale manufacturing of ultra-high viscosity alginates of clinical-grade, the development of highly sensitive *in vitro* assays for screening of apoptotic and mitogenic impurities, as well as the improvement of the alginate cross-linking process can be considered as important steps towards the clinical realization of the concepts of alginate-based cell therapy and tissue regeneration. However, long-term transplantation studies in small and large animal models are required before medical approval of these novel alginate microcapsules can be granted and clinical applications can then be envisaged. The quality of the algal material is crucial for the production of large-scale clinical-grade alginates. The apoptosis assay is very rapid and efficient, both from the medical and economical point of view (compared to transplantation in BB rats). It can be used to prove the quality of the algal material during harvesting, but also for routine validation of the individual steps of the extraction and purification process of alginate. For clinical application long-term storage of validated grafts is an additional important pre-requisite and has been neglected hitherto. Cryoconservation was not possible to date because of the high water content of the alginate and the incomplete cross-linking process. The crystal gun method, together with recent progress in the formulation of cryoprotecting agents and proteins [12], will most likely overcome this problem.

References

1. Bedner E, Li X, Gorczyca W, Melamed MR, Darzynkiewicz Z (1999) Analysis of apoptosis by laser scanning cytometry. Cytometry 35:181–195
2. Diamond DA, Caldamone AA (1999) Endoscopic correction of vesicoureteral reflux in children using autologous chondrocytes: preliminary results. J Urol 162:1185–1188
3. Dornish M, Kaplan D, Skaugrud O (2001) Standards and guidelines for biopolymers in tissue-engineered medical products: ASTM alginate and chitosan standard guides. American Society for Testing and Materials. Ann N Y Acad Sci 944:388–397
4. Geisen K, Deutschländer H, Gorbach S, Klenke C, Zimmermann U (1990) Function of barium-alginate microencapsulated xenogenic islets in different diabetic mouse models. In: Shafrir E (ed) Frontiers in diabetes research. Lessons from animal diabetes III. Smith-Gordon, London, pp142–148
5. Hasse C, Klöck G, Schlosser A, Zimmermann U, Rothmund M (1997) Parathyroid allotransplantation without immunosuppression. Lancet 350:1296–1297
6. Hillgärtner M, Zimmermann H, Mimietz S et al. (1999) Immunoisolation of transplants by entrapment in 19F-labelled alginate gels: production, biocompatibility, stability, and long-term monitoring of functional integrity. Mat-Wiss Werkstofftech 30:783–792
7. Hoffman AS (2001) Hydrogels for biomedical applications. Ann N Y Acad Sci 944:62–73
8. Hunkeler D, Cherrington A, Prokop A, Rajotte R (2001) Bioartificial organs III. Tissue sourcing, immunoisolation and clinical trials. The New York Academy of Sciences, New York
9. Kühtreiber WM, Lanza RP, Chick WL (1999) Cell encapsulation technology and therapeutics. Birkhäuser, Boston
10. Leinfelder U, Brunnenmeier F, Cramer H, Schiller J, Arnold K, Vásquez JA, Zimmermann U (2003) A highly sensitive cell assay for validation of purification regimes of alginates (submitted)
11. Schneider S, Feilen P, Cramer H, Hillgärtner M, Brunnenmeier F, Zimmermann H, Zimmermann U (2003) Beneficial effects of human serum albumin on stability and functionality of alginate microcapsules fabricated in different ways (submitted)
12. Shirakashi R, Köstner CM, Müller KJ, Kürschner M, Zimmermann U, Sukhorukov VL (2002) Intracellular delivery of trehalose into mammalian cells by electropermeabilization. J Memb Biol 189:45–54
13. Smiley ST, Reers M, Mottola-Hartshorn C et al. (1991) Intracellular heterogeneity in mitochondrial membrane potentials revealed by a J-aggregate-forming lipophilic cation JC-1. Proc Natl Acad Sci 88:3671–3675
14. Weber M, Steinert A, Jork A, Dimmler A, Thürmer F, Schütze N, Hendrich C, Zimmermann U (2002) Formation of cartilage matrix proteins by BMP-transfected murine mesenchymal stem cells encapsulated in a novel class of alginates. Biomaterials 23:2003–2013
15. Zimmermann U, Klöck G, Federlin K et al. (1992) Production of mitogen-contamination free alginates with variable ratios of mannuronic acid to guluronic acid by free flow electrophoresis. Electrophoresis 13:269–274
16. Zimmermann H, Hagedorn R, Richter E, Fuhr G (1999a) Topography of cell traces studied by atomic force microscopy. Eur Biophys 28:516–525
17. Zimmermann U, Hasse C, Rothmund M, Kühtreiber W (1999b) Biocompatible encapsulation materials: fundamentals and application. In: Kühtreiber WM, Lanza RP, Chick WL (eds) Cell encapsulation technology and therapeutics. Birkhäuser, Boston, pp40–52
18. Zimmermann, U, Mimietz S, Zimmermann H et al. (2000) Hydrogel-based non-autologous cell and tissue therapy. Biotechniques 29:564–581
19. Zimmermann U, Thürmer F, Jork A et al. (2001a) A novel class of amitogenic alginate microcapsules for long-term immunoisolated transplantation. Ann N Y Acad Sci 944:199–215
20. Zimmermann U, Cramer H, Jork A et al. (2001b) Microencapsulation-based cell therapy. In: Reed G, Rehm HJ (eds) Biotechnology. Wiley-VCH, Weinheim, pp547–571
21. Zimmermann H, Hillgärtner M, Manz B et al. (2003) Fabrication of homogeneously cross-linked, functional alginate microcapsules validated by NMR-, CLSM- and AFM-imaging. Biomaterials (in press)

CHAPTER 10

Collagen and Hyaluronic Acid   **10**

Hartmut F. Hildebrand and Nicolas Blanchemain

Introduction

Cartilage is a specialized connective tissue, which is solid, elastic, compact, and flexible. It is essential for the movement of joints and has an important role during bone development. The embryonic skeleton is constituted of cartilage, which is replaced during growth to bone, except in some parts of the joints, ribs, larynx, respiratory tract, and the maxillo-facial region.

Cartilage is considered an avascular connective tissue. However, Peyron and Stanescu [23] have reported the presence of vascular channels in the deep layers of articular cartilage suggesting hat these capillaries are important for nutrition and oxygen supply. Recently, cartilage has found an increasing interest in tissue engineering for 4 reasons:

- culture of autologous chondrocytes for re-implantation in patients and repair of articular cartilage defects [1, 3, 4, 13, 17],
- integration of chondrocytes in collagen and hyaluronic acid gels and waxes for esthetic and plastic surgery [28],
- preparation of biodegradable devices for drug delivery systems [24], and
- development of scaffold materials and hybrid biomaterials [17, 20, 21, 27].

Different Cartilage Forms

Cartilage is composed of a matrix of hydrophilic proteins, proteoglycans, and glucoseoaminoglycans (GAGs) integrated in a network of collagen fibers. The matrix serves as a support for chondrocytes, which have both anabolic and catabolic activities [11]. The chondrocytes not only synthesize the extracellular matrix, but also the enzymes for matrix degradation. The most common GAGs are chondroitin sulfate, keratane sulfate, and hyaluronic acid (HA). The latter is composed partially of glucoseamines. The proteoglycans bind water and cations to form a viscous and elastic layer with lubricant and shock absorbing functions. The overall composition of cartilage is given in Fig. 10.1. Water is the main component with 70% to 80%. The cellular component is 8% to 12%. Important variations exist between the cartilage types and the different cartilage sites [10]. The different composition defines 3 types of cartilage each with specific histological features, due to the presence of different collagen types and variations of the extracellular matrix [15].

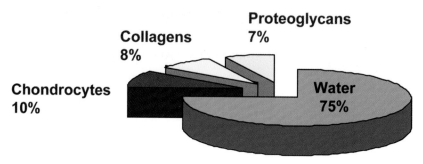

Fig. 10.1. Distribution of the main components of cartilage.

Hyaline cartilage is characterized by a homogenous extracellular matrix containing mostly collagen type II fibers. The matrix forms multiple lacunae containing mostly 2 to 3 chondrocytes. This type is surrounded by a perichondrium. The hyaline cartilage is located in the "C"-rings in the trachea, the nose, and in particular at the articular ends of bones. In the adult its function is mainly the support of the soft tissue, lubricant, and shock absorption in joints.

The matrix of the *elastic cartilage* is characterized by abundant elastic fibers, which can be easily seen under light microscopy. These fibers give great flexibility to the tissue. Two or 3 chondrocytes are embedded in lacunae similar to hyaline cartilage. This type is also surrounded by a perichondrium. Its main location is in the ear, the auditory canal, and the epiglottis. The main function is to give flexible support to the soft tissue.

Fibrocartilage is recognized by the specific orientation of the chondrocytes in rows. Lacunae, which lodge the chondrocytes in the other cartilage types are not visible. The specific structure of the matrix is due to the numerous nearly parallelorganized collagen fibers, giving the tissue the characteristic durability. Fibrocartilage has no perichondrium. This type is found in the pubic symphysis and is the fundamental substance of the intervertebral disc. It has the highest amount of HA. Its function is to support soft and hard tissue and in particular to withstand compression.

Matrix Molecules of Cartilage

The 3 main components of cartilage are chondrocytes, a network of collagen fibers, and proteoglycans.

Collagens

The cartilage collagens are mainly synthesized and secreted by chondroblasts and in lower amounts by osteoblasts and fibroblasts. The principal collagen in all forms of cartilage is collagen type II [27]. Other types have been identified and their distribution and function has been investigated:

- Collagen type IX is normally associated with articular cartilage and its preferential site is the cartilage surface beneath the perichondrium.
- Low amounts of collagen types VI and XI have been described.
- Collagen types V and X are existing in some specific cartilage types (contamination with serum collagens and the appearance related to pathological defects has to be clarified).

There is nearly no collagen "turn-over" in cartilage, which could explain the very limited possibilities of repair.

Hyaluronic Acid (HA)

HA is a fundamental substance of any connective tissue. It is synthesized and secreted by multiple cell types, in particular by chondrocytes, fibroblasts and synoviocytes. Its main distribution site is cartilage, with a significant high specificity for fibrocartilage. HA is also found in synovial fluids. Combined to soluble collagens it is present in all body fluids, e.g. in serum, lymphatic liquid, and in the aqueous and vitreous fluid of the eye. Therefore, it is currently used as a visco-elastic agent in eye surgery.

HA is fabricated as gels, waxes, scaffolds, and other forms of implant materials by different methods. The most frequent technique is the extraction and purification from cockscomb. Modern techniques allow preparing synthetic HA via genetic recombination or directly *in vitro*. The main role of HA is to assume the mechanical function as a lubricant of cartilage and joints. Chondrocytes produce HA as their own extracellular matrix, and subsequently as their own support, but these cells also synthesize the degradation enzymes of HA, and thus assure its continuous turnover and renewing under normal physiological conditions [6, 9]. This physiological dual role gives a better understanding of the metabolic interactions with chondrocytes, synoviocytes, leukocytes, and nociceptors [11]. HA is a high molecular weight polysaccharide from the GAG family. The basic molecule is a polymer of the repeated disaccharide unit composed of the D-glucuronic acid and N-acetyl-D-glucoseamine (Fig. 10.2A).

Other Glucoseaminoglycans

Other GAGs, which are mainly found associated with HA are:
- glucoseaminosulfate (a polymer of a aminomonosaccharide),
- chondroitin sulfate (a polymer of the repeated disaccharide unit composed of the alternant D-glucuronic acid and N-acetyl-D-galactoseamine sulfate; Fig. 10.2B)
- keratane sulfate (a polymer of a repeated disaccharide unit composed of the alternant galactose and N-acetyl-glucoseamine-6-sulfate; Fig. 10.2C).

Together with HA, as a central molecule, all these GAGs form a highly visco-elastic proteoglycan, which retains water and cations (Fig. 10.3) [17].

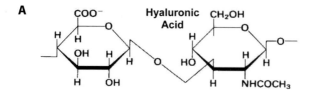

A   Hyaluronic Acid

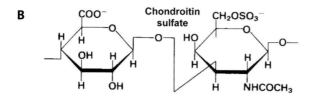

B   Chondroitin sulfate

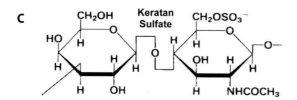

C   Keratan Sulfate

Fig. 10.2A–C. Chemical formula of hyaluronic acid (**A**), chondroitin sulfate (**B**) and keratane sulfate (**C**).

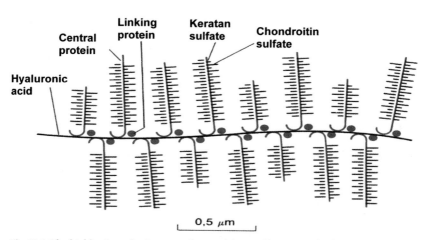

Fig. 10.3. The highly visco-elastic proteoglycan of the cartilage ground substance with hyaluronic acid as central molecule.

The Role of HA in Cartilage Degradation and Healing

The concentration and molecular weight and therefore the molecular chain length of HA are reduced in arthritis. This implies the decrease of the visco-elastic quality of cartilage and induces the perturbation of the proteoglycan synthesis. A complementation of HA, with respect to its extremely low immune and inflammatory reactions, has therapeutic functions in the treatment of arthritis [6, 9, 25], wound healing (application of gels and waxes) [7, 13], and in skin diseases [18]. Combined to collagen it is used in plastic surgery [28] for the treatment of wrinkles, skin folds, filling of larger tissue areas, and as scaffold for tissue engineered implants [17, 21]. The application is only temporary because of the degradation of both, HA and collagen. HA dissolves within 7 to 8 months, collagens dissolve within 6 to 8 months. Combinations of both may "survive" up to 18 months under optimal conditions, such as improvement of the biopolymer reticulation by de-polymerization/re-polymerization processes [14, 22]. The degradation of cartilage is mechanical and physiological [9, 25]. The implied enzymes are hyaluronidase and collagenase. Mechanical stress can induce physiological effects on chondrocyte metabolism and inhibit or decrease the HA and collagen synthesis.

The Use of HA and Collagens as Medical Devices

It is well known that articular cartilage tissue has a very low capacity to regenerate because of its missing vascularization. If damaged, the cartilage is replaced by a fibrocartilage, containing mostly collagen type I, without sufficient function compared to normal intact articular cartilage [29]. Therefore, gels, waxes, porous scaffolds, and composite matrices have been developed. HA and collagen scaffolds have to fulfill two principle features: support for tissue engineered implants/hybrid biomaterials and stimulation of the physiological mechanisms, such as growth factor signaling and integration of different cell types [7, 12, 17].

Fabrication of Scaffolds

The main problem in the fabrication of HA and collagen composite matrices is the formation of polyion complexes (PICs), i.e. heterogenous matrices in aqueous solutions due to their opposite electrostatical charges. Different methods have been developed and evaluated to optimize conditions that PICs are is not formed between HA and collagen type II. One of these conditions is the direct cross-linking using the water-soluble carbodiimide WSC [1-ethyl-3-(3-dimethyl aminopropyl) carbodiimide hydrochloride] [27]. HA-collagen composite matrices were successfully obtained using WSC in the presence of 0.4 M NaCl, which was found the optimal concentration to suppress PIC formation. In addition, the swelling ratio of the HA-collagen matrix was directly influenced by the concentration of HA. Scanning electron microscopy (SEM) revealed the multipore structure of the lyophilized matrices.

While HA has been shown to influence the swelling capacity of HA-scaffolds, WSC has a dose-dependent action on the collagenase activity. In enzymatic degradation tests WSC treated HA-collagen scaffolds and membranes showed significant enhancement of the resistance to collagenase activity, in comparison with glutaraldehyde treated matrices. The freeze drying temperature (–20 °C, –70 °C, and –196 °C) has also an influence on the pore size, varying with mean diameters of 230, 90, and 40 μm, respectively. The porosity of 58% to 65% is also related to the applied freeze drying temperature [21]. All variations of pore size, porosity, and resistance to collagenase degradation are independent from the cross-linking degree. Cytotoxicity tests with mouse fibroblasts cultured in, or on the scaffolds or membranes, revealed no significant toxicity of the WSC-cross-linked matrices.

In Vitro Engineering of Cartilage

Studies were performed to design biosystems containing embedded chondrocytes to fill osteochondral defects and to produce a tissue substitute close to native cartilage. An interesting alternative to HA-collagen matrices are HA-alginate sponges [20]. Large-porosity sponges were obtained through freeze-dried sodium alginate solutions with or without HA. This formulation was compared with a hydrogel of the same composition. In the sponge formulation, macroscopic and microscopic studies demonstrated the formation of associated macro-porous and micro-porous networks, with an average pore size of 175 μm and 250 nm, respectively. Histological and biochemical analysis showed, that when loaded with HA, the sponge provides an adapted environment for proteoglycan and collagen synthesis by chondrocytes. Cytoskeleton assessment by three-dimensional fluorescence microscopy revealed a marked spherical shape of chondrocytes with non-orientated and sparse actin microfilaments. In addition, collagen type I was detected in both types of sponges (with or without HA). These sponges open new perspectives in tissue engineering for the *in vitro* fabrication of "artificial" cartilage. Furthermore, the presence of HA within the alginate sponge mimics a functional environment suitable for the synthesis and secretion of extracellular matrix by embedded chondrocytes.

Effects of HA on Chondrocyte Activity

Synthesized and secreted by chondrocytes, HA acts in normal cartilage by a feedback mechanism with a significant influence on chondrocyte proliferation and subsequently on glucoseamine synthesis [3, 4, 13, 17]. Multiple *in vitro* studies have been performed to determine the chondrocyte activity [17, 21]. A successful scaffold respects and assures these activities. Kawasaki et al. [17] have demonstrated that this challenge can be obtained by different compounds normally contained in healthy cartilage. For these purposes they have isolated chondrocytes from rabbit articular cartilage, which were cultured in collagen gels with various amounts of HA for 4 weeks. Morphological and histological studies demonstrated that HA-treated chondrocytes in collagen gels proliferated and maintained their phenotype. At post-culture week 4 the addition of 0.1 mg/mL HA induced an 8-fold increase in cell number compared to HA-pretreatment values. Synthesis of chondroitin 6-sulfate in groups treated with 0.01 and 0.1 mg/mL HA significantly increased, while gel accumulation rates in groups treated with 0.1 and 1.0 mg/mL of HA showed significantly higher values. The authors clearly demonstrated, that in collagen gel cultures HA enhanced the proliferation and the chondroitin 6-sulfate synthesis, while maintaining their phenotype. It should be emphasized that this *in vitro* model could be a suitable model for clinical applications. Since the supply of autologous chondrocytes for transplantation is not unlimited [1, 3, 4, 13] the HA-treated culture method may be useful for increasing the number of active chondrocytes and thus improving the quality of implants and hybrid medical devices.

Effects of HA on Fibroblast Activity

Similar experiments were performed to assess the fibroblast activity in collagen matrix for improvement of dermal wound healing [7, 12]. After suspending human dermal fibroblasts in a collagen matrix they showed a 4-day delay in cell division, while the same cells in monolayer culture divided by day 1. Proliferation rates were assessed by ^{3}H-thymidine incorporation. The initial rates of incorporation by cells of both culture systems were not significantly different. When suspended in collagen, there was a 3-fold increase in the proportion of cells in a tetraploid (4N) DNA state compared to cells in monolayer cultures. Flow cytometry analysis and ^{3}H-thymidine incorporation studies identified the delay of cell division as a consequence of a block in the G2/M phase of the cell cycle and not an inhibition of DNA synthesis.

The inclusion of 150 µg/mL of HA in the production of fibroblast populated collagen lattice (FPCL) [2] caused a stimulation of cell division, an increased expression of tubulin, and a reduction the proportion of cells in the 4N state. HA added to the same cells growing in monolayer, showed a very little increase in the rate of cell division or DNA synthesis. HA supplementation of FPCLs stimulated cell division, as well as tubulin concentrations, but did not enhance lattice contraction. Supported by other experimental series, the authors come to the conclusion that at least in human fibroblasts suspended in collagen gels the effect of HA could stimulate the synthesis of tubulin. Suh and Lee have also confirmed the regenerative potential of HA on dermal fibroblasts under different experimental conditions [26].

Conclusion

The etiology of degenerative articular diseases is multifactorial. Mechanical reasons are the most cited in clinical case reports [16]. The degeneration of articular cartilage is a frequent reason for pain and invalidity of elderly people. Articular cartilage is a complex structure with a very limited capacity for repair [9]. When a cartilage trauma goes deeply into the subchondral bone it produces bone marrow cell migration into the lesion. This phenomenon is accompanied by a inflammatory reaction leading to the formation of fibrocartilage [16]. The correlation of age, frequency of arthritis, and alterations of chondrocyte function suggests that trauma plays a critical role in the onset of osteoarthritis [5]. The response of articular cartilage to acute (trauma) or chronic (degenerative) injury is an imperfect repair. The mechanical and biochemical properties of the repair tissue differ from the original cartilage, resulting in a functional deficit [8]. Currently different surgical techniques for articular cartilage repair are in clinical use. The results of these procedures differ. Only the transplantation of osteochondral grafts can restore articular cartilage with a true hyalin-like repair tissue. But this technique is limited because of donor site limitations.

Most cartilage-specific macromolecules have been extensively used for therapeutic application in form of isolated or combined injections. Clinical and experimental studies with chondrocytes have confirmed the advantage of HA as a surgical aid in ophthalmology, joint disease, arthritis, wound healing, and skin disease. Bound to collagen it is currently used in plastic surgery and many patients are grateful using collagen-HA composites, providing them with smooth skin, due to the reduction of wrinkles and folds. The functional potentials also show the importance of HA for the fabrication of scaffolds, gels, waxes, sponges, and other porous or dense composite matrices. For the repair of articular cartilage many researchers have performed studies using different combinations of collagens, alginates, glucoseamines, GAGs, and proteoglycans. Among these, HA is certainly of high importance and could be beneficial because of its multiple functional potentials and qualities. HA increases the swelling ratio and conditions the porous structure. It regulates the interaction between different cell types and stimulates chondrocyte and fibroblast proliferation by increasing tubulin synthesis and controlling the diploid DNA state. Furthermore, it enhances chondroitin sulfate synthesis in chondrocytes. In the future, additional potential applications of HA for therapeutic and diagnostic means will be developed and increase the importance of that omnipresent macromolecule in the human organism.

References

1. Aston JE, Bentley G (1986) Repair of articular surfaces by allografts of articular and growth-plate cartilage. J Bone Joint Surg-Br 69:29–35
2. Bell E, Ivarsson B, Merrill C (1979) Production of a tissue like structure by contraction of collagen lattices by human fibroblasts of different proliferative potential *in vitro*. Proc Natl Acad Sci 76:1274–1278
3. Brittberg M, Lindahl A, Nilsson A, Ohlsson A, Isaksson O, Peterson L (1994) Treatment of deep cartilage defects treated with autologous chondrocyte transplantation. N Engl J Med 331:889–895
4. Brittberg M, Nilsson A, Lindahl A, Ohlsson A, Peterson L (1996) Rabbit articular cartilage defects treated with autologous cultured chondrocyte. Clin Orthop 326:1270–1283
5. Buckwalter JA, Mankin AJ (1998) Articular cartilage: degeneration and osteoarthitis, repair, regeneration, and transplantation. Instr Course Lect 47:487–504
6. Chen FS, Frenkel SR, Di Cesare PE (1999) Repair of articular cartilage defects: part I. Basic Science of cartilage healing. Am J Orthop 28:31–33
7. Doillon CJ, Silver FH (1986) Collagen-based wound dressing: effects of Hyaluronic acid and fibronectin on wound healing. Biomaterials 7:3–8
8. Frenkel SR, Di Cesare PE (1999) Degradation and repair of articular cartilage. Front Biosci 15:671–685
9. Ghivizzani SC, Oligino TJ, Robbins PD, Evans CH (2000) Cartilage injury and repair. Phys Med Rehabil Clin N Am 11:289–307
10. Goa KL, Bryson HM (1994) Hyaluronic acid: a review of its pharmacology and use as a surgical aid in ophthalmology, and its therapeutic potential in joint disease and wound healing. Drugs 47:536–566
11. Goto H, Onodera T, Hirano H, Shimamura T (1999) Hyaluronic acid suppression caused by interleukin-1beta in cultured rabbit articular chondrocytes. Tohoku J Exp Med 187:1–13
12. Greco RM, Iocono JA, Ehrlich HP (1998) Hyaluronic acid stimulates human fibroblast proliferation within a collagen matrix. J Cell Physiol 177:465–473

13. Green WT Jr (1977) Articular cartilage repair: behavior of rabbit chondrocytes during tissue culture and subsequent allografting. Clin Orthop 124:237–250
14. Hildebrand HF, Rocher P, Monchau F, Delcourt-Debruyne E (2002) Kollagen: Aufbereitung und Eigenschaften als Biomaterial. Biomaterialien 3:14–20
15. Histology of cartilage: http://www.usc.edu/hsc/dental/ghisto/index.html
16. Imhof H, Breitenseher M, Kainberger F, Trattnig S (1997) Degenerative joint disease: cartilage or vascular disease? Skeletal Radiol 26:398–403
17. Kawasaki K, Ochi M, Uchio Y, Adachi N, Matsusaki M (1999) Hyaluronic acid enhances proliferation and chondroitin sulfate synthesis in cultured chondrocytes embedded in collagen gels. J Cell Physiol 179:142–148
18. Konohana A, Miyakawa S, Tajima S, Nishikawa T (1986) Decreased collagen and hyaluronic acid content in lesional skin of acrogeria. Dermatologica 172:241–244
19. Lodish H, Darnell J, Baltimore D (1989) La cellule biologie moléculaire. Editions Vigot, Paris, pp97–100
20. Miralles R, Baudoin R, Dumas D et al. (2000) Sodium alginate sponges with or without sodium hyaluronate: In vitro engineering of cartilage. J Biomed Mater Res 57:568–278
21. Park SN, Park JC, Kim HO, Song MJ, Suh H (2002) Characterization of porous collagen/hyaluronic acid scaffold modified by 1-ethyl-3-(3-dimethylaminopropyl)carbodiimide cross linking. Biomaterials 23:1205–1212
22. Petite H, Rault I, Huc A, Menache PH, Herbage D (1990) Use of the azyl-azide method for cross-linking collagen rich tissues such as pericardium. J Biomed Mat Res 24:179–187
23. Peyron J, Stanescu V (1994) Cartilage articulaire normal de l'adulte. Anatomie, physiologie, métabolisme, vieillissement. Editions Techniques, Encycl Méd Chim, Paris. Appareil locomoteur, 14–003-A-10 pp14
24. Prestwitch GD, Marecak DM, Marecek JF, Vercruysse KP, Ziebell MR (1998) Controlled chemical modification of hyaluronic acid: synthesis, applications and biodegradation of hydrazyde derivatives. J Controlled Rel 53:93–103
25. Setton LA, Elliott DM, Mow VC (1999) Altered mechanics of cartilage with osteoarthritis: human osteoarthritis and an experimental model of joint degeneration. Osteoarthritis Cartilage 7:2–14
26. Suh H, Lee JE (2002) Behavior of fibroblasts on a porous hyaluronic acid incorporated collagen matrix. Yonsei Med J 43:193–202
27. Taguchi T, Ikoma T, Tanaka J (2002) An improved method to prepare hyaluronic acid and type II collagen composite matrices. J Biomed Mater Res 61:330–336
28. Taguchi T, Tanaka J (2002) Swelling behavior of hyaluronic acid and type II collagen hydrogels prepared by using conventional crosslinking and subsequent additional polymer interactions. J Biomater Sci Polym Ed 13:43–52
29. Temenoff JS, Mikos AG (2000) Review: tissue engineering for regeneration of articular cartilage. Biomaterials 21:431–440

CHAPTER 11

Biodegradable Polymers 11

HANS PISTNER

Introduction

Biological polymers have been used for hundreds of years as medical devices such as ligatures (Susruta/India 500 b.C., Galen 2nd century a.C.). Lister in 1868 introduced "animal tissue" for wound closure [31]. Heine (1878), Socin (1879), and Gluck (1891) implanted ivory for the induction of new bone formation and the healing of bone gaps [20, 21, 54]. Today such procedures are summarized as "tissue engineering techniques". In the 50's the idea to use polymers made from physiological substrates for tissue adaptation and as scaffold materials came up. Beside collagens, which today are widely used for different indications, polylactic acid (PLA) and polyglycolic acid (PGA) were the first substrates used.

Polylactic acid (PLA)

Lactic acid in its impure form has been detected in 1780 by the Swedish chemist Scheele [50]. In 1932 Carothers and co-workers first succeeded in polymerization, creating a resinous substance [9]. Ring-opening polymerization of dilactide (Lowe, Klein, Trustee, Ditch) gave results with much higher molecular weight and better mechanical properties [32]. Polymers of pure Poly-L-Lactide (PLLA; Fig. 11.1) develop a helical structure [11] and are able to crystalize to a high degree [3].

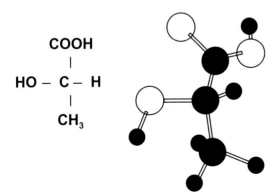

COOH
|
HO – C – H
|
CH₃

Fig. 11.1.
Illustration of PLLA.

The polymer is hydrolyzed in an aqueous environment to lactic acid and metabolized via the citric acid cycle (Fig. 11.2).

These highly crystaline substances were soon used for osteosyntheses. They proved to be biodegradable but not bioresorbable [38] and induced a late inflammatory tissue response [4, 36]. Amorphous PLLA of different molecular weight, produced by injection molding, showed resorption according to the 4 stages described by Kronenthal [28] (Table 11.1), without a clinical relevant inflammation [39–41].

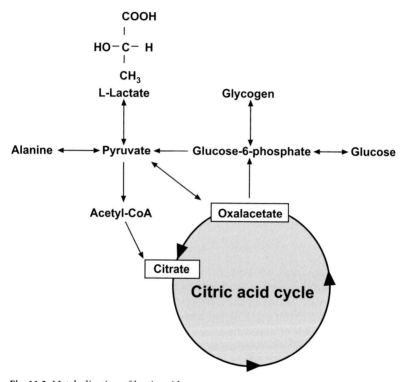

Fig. 11.2. Metabolization of lactic acid.

Table 11.1. Stages of polymer degradation according to Krohnenthal (1975)

Stage	Procedure	Origin and cause
1	Hydratation	Loosening of van der Waals forces and hydrogen bridging forces
2	Loss of stability	Initial fission of covalent chemical bonds of the backbone
3	Loss of form	Further fission of covalent chemical bonds Molecular weight becomes insufficient for coherence
4	Loss of mass	Dissolution of low molecular compounds Phagozytosis of small fragments

Polyglycolic Acid (PGA)

Glycolic acid is the chemical more simple variation of lactic acid. A hydrogen molecule replaces the hydrophobic methyl-group (CH_3) in the lactic acid molecule. Therefore, all polymers containing glycolic acid are more hydrophilic and faster degradable by hydrolization (Fig. 11.3).

Bischoff and co-workers first described this compound in 1893 [5]. The synthesis is similar to polylactides via the dimer [9]. Following hydrolysis PGA is partly excreted through the kidneys. It is metabolized via glyoxylate, glycine, and to lactic acid and becomes a substrate of the citric acid cycle. Glycolic acid compounds are widely used as suture materials and for osteosynthesis. Again, in many cases osteolytic and inflammatory tissue response occurs.

Polydioxanone

Another compound in clinical use is polydioxanone (Fig. 11.4). In contrast to polyglycolides it has a carbonyl group substituted by 2 hydrogen atoms. Therefore, it is less hydrophilic and degrades slower than polyglycolides. Degradation and metabolization are not sufficiently analyzed [45]. Nevertheless, it is used for resorbable suture materials and in part for low-load bearing osteosyntheses [8, 15, 16, 18, 19, 35, 58].

Trimethylencarbonate

By co-polymerization of 32.5% trimethylencarbonate with 67.5% glycolic acid the raw material for sutures with similar behavior as polydioxanone was created [47].

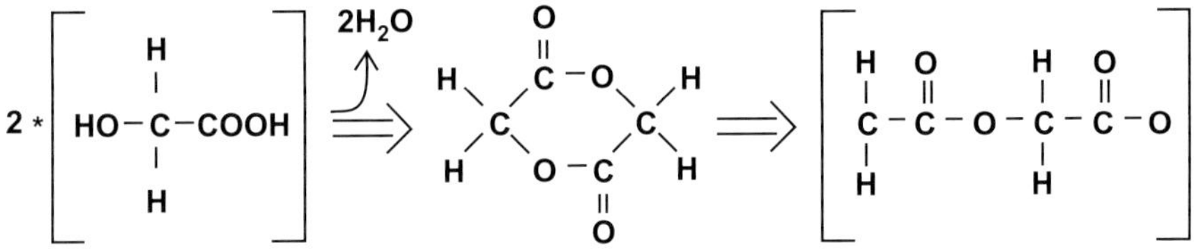

Fig. 11.3. Illustration of the structure and synthesis of PGA.

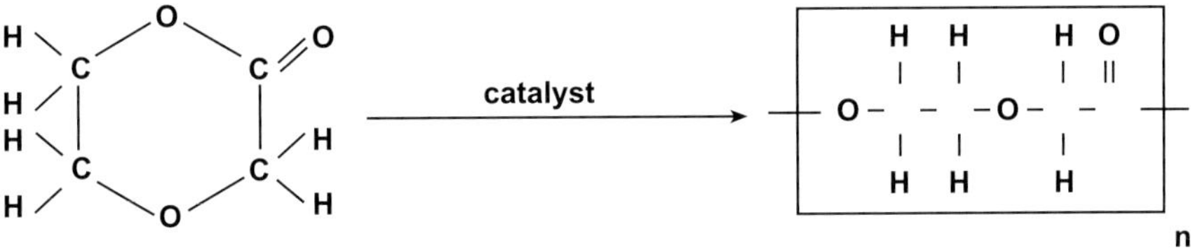

Fig. 11.4. Illustration of structure and synthesis of polydioxanone.

Resorption within 200 to 300 days was shown by Knoop and co-workers 1987 [26] (Fig. 11.5).

Polyhydroxybutyrate

This compound is characterized by the addition of a CH_2-group to the lactic acid monomer [1]. Therefore, it is less hydrophilic compared to polylactide. Again, full resorption has not been proved [22, 29] (Fig. 11.6).

Polyhydroxyvalerate

Adding another CH_2-group to the side chain of the monomer will result in polyhydroxyvalerate. This substance has been co-polymerized with polyhydroxybutyrate (Biopol®) [6] (Fig. 11.7).

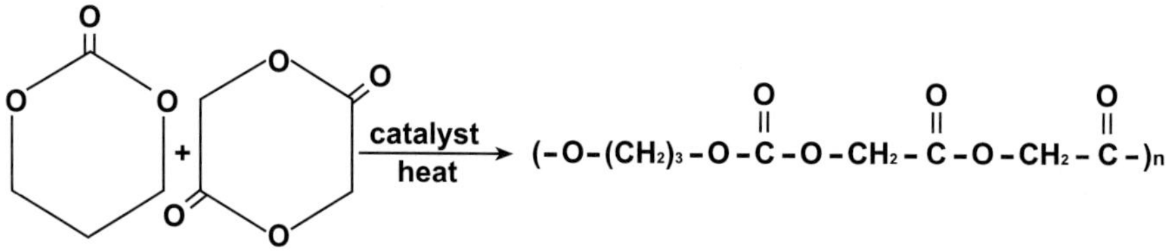

Fig. 11.5. Illustration of structure and synthesis of trimethylene-glycolide-copolymer (MaxonR).

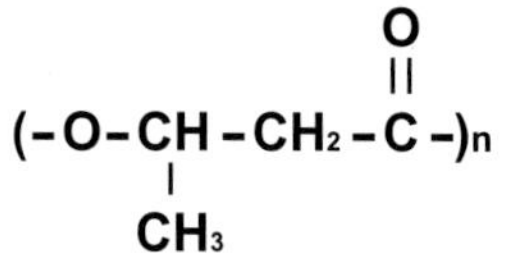

Fig. 11.6. Illustration of the structure of polyhydroxybutyrate.

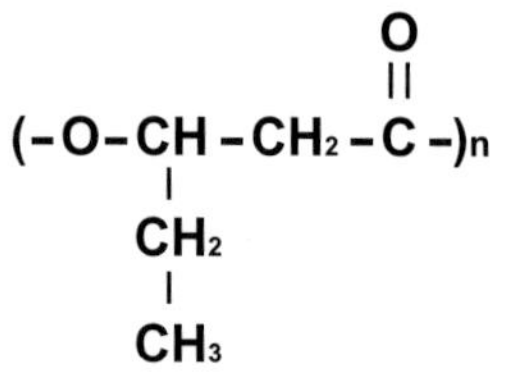

Fig. 11.7. Illustration of the structure of polyhydroxyvalerate.

Polycaprolactone

ε-caprolactone is a ring-forming compound such as lactide, glycolide, and para-diox-anone. By ring-opening polymerization polycaprolactone is synthesized from this compound. It degrades *in vivo* very slowly [44]. Fragments are resorbed via intracellular enzymatic degradation by phagocytes [57]. It has been tested for sutures, fibers, and as a drug delivery material [43, 53] (Fig. 11.8).

Other Candidates

Many other compounds are candidates for different clinical purposes. Most of them are less characterized. More than 1000 publications since the year 1990 has made it difficult to give a complete overview. The following list gives examples of other candidates:

- oligo(α-hydroxycarbonacid)acrylate-copolymer [34],
- polyanhydride [30],
- polycarbonate [10],
- polyesteramide [2],
- polyethylencarbonate [24],
- polyethylenoxid-polylactide-copolymer [59],
- polyiminocarbonate [27],
- polyorthoester [17]
- polyphosphate/polyphosphonate [46]

Biodegradable or Bioresorbable?

It is important to ask if a so-called biodegradable biomaterial will show tissue reaction in the long run [37]. If this is the case it is mostly due to the so-called "particle disease". This means that the materials are biodegraded to a critical size and macrophages will take up the resulting particles. If it is not possible for the macrophage to degrade and dissolve these particles, e. g. enzymatically, the macrophages will die and the cell debris including the particles will initiate a vitious circle, resulting in a clinical relevant inflammation. This process has been described after implantation of temporo-mandibluar joint prostheses [14] and hip prostheses [33], and it might also be

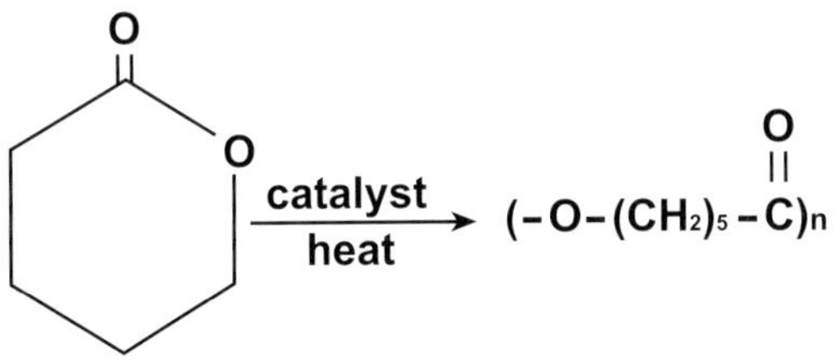

Fig. 11.8.
Illustration of structure and synthesis of polycaprolactone.

true for the so-called "biodegradable materials". In contrast, bioresorbable compounds like amorphous polylactides do not induce a clinical relevant inflammation and are of high value for tissue engineering applications.

Conclusion

Resorbable polymers are the ideal materials for *in situ* tissue induction and "guided tissue regeneration". The essential idea is to create structures which have the exact shape of the body part to be reconstructed. For instance, this might be a peace of missing bone. The structure must consist of a resorbable substance and should be strong enough to stabilize the surrounding tissues, ideally like a metal plate for osteosynthesis. These constructs can be loaded with morphogens or signaling substances, which can be delivered to the site of new tissue growth [42]. Today this is still a vision, but in reconstructive surgery the guided tissue regeneration concept allows nerve fibers to grow through resorbable tubes replacing autologous nerve transplantation [51]. The concept of *in situ* tissue induction will facilitate procedures, which could replace cells by morphogens and will make *in situ* tissue engineering affordable for many applications in medicine.

References

1. Baptist J, Ziegler J (1965) Method of making absorbable surgical sutures from poly beta hydroxy acids. US-Patent 3 225 766, 28
2. Barrows T, Grussing D, Hegdahl D (1983) Poly(Ester-Amides): A new class of synthetic absorbable polymers. Trans Soc Biomat 6:109
3. Bendix D (1990) Changes in the molecular weight distribution of amorphous and crystalline poly(l-lactide) during degradation in vivo. 7th Meeting of the European Society of Biomechanics, Aarhus, Denmark, July 8–11, 1990
4. Bergsma E, Rozema F, Bos R, De Bruijn W (1993) Foreign body reactions to resorbable poly(l-lactide) bone plates and screws used for the fixation of unstable zygomatic fractures. J Oral Maxillofac Surg 51:666–670
5. Bischoff C, Walden P (1893) Glycolids and its homologs. Ber 26:262–265
6. Bluhm T, Hamer G, Marchessault R, Fyfe C, Veregin R (1986) Morphology of a novel copolyester: bacterial poly(β-hydroxybutyrate-co-β-hydroxyvalerate). Polm Prepr 27:250–251
7. Böstmann O(1991) Osteolytic changes accompanying degradation of absorbable fracture implants. J Bone Joint Surg-Br 73:679–682
8. Bucher H (1984) Absorbierbare Osteosyntheseschrauben aus Polydioxanon (PDS) im Tierexperiment. Thesis, Universität Würzburg
9. Carothers W, Dorough G, Van Natta F (1932) Studies of polymerization and ring formation; X. The reversible polymerization of six-membered cyclic esters. J Am Chem Soc 54:761–772
10. Choueka J, Charvet J, Koval K et al. (1996) Canine bone response to tyrosine-derived polycarbonates and poly(l-lactic acid). J Biomed Mater Res 31:35–41
11. De Santis P, Kovacs A (1968) Molecular conformation of poly(s-lactic acid). Biopolymers 6:299–306
12. Dittrich W, Schulz R (1971) Kinetik und Mechanismus der ringöffnenden Polymerisation von L-Lactid. Angew Makromol Chem 15:109–126
13. Doddi N u. Versfeld C (1977) Synthetic absorbable surgical devices of polydioxanone. U.S.-Patent No. 40 422 988
14. Dolwick M, Aufdemorte T (1985) Silicone-induced foreign body reaction and lymphadenopathy after temporomandibular joint arthroplasty. Oral Surg Oral Med Oral Pathol 59:449–452

15. Dumbach J (1984) Zugschraubenosteosynthese nach Ramus-Osteotomie mit resorbierbaren Osteosyntheseschrauben aus Polydioxanon (PDS). – Erste Ergebnisse. Dtsch Z Mund Kiefer GesichtsChir 8:145–148
16. Dumbach J (1987) Osteosynthese mit resorbierbaren PDS-Stiften nach sagittaler Spaltung und Rückversetzung des Unterkiefers. Dtsch Zahnärztl Z 42:9–12
17. Ekholm M, Syrjänen S, Laine P, Lindquist C, Kellomäki M, Virtanen I, Ruuronen R (1966) Biocompatibility of solid poly(orthoester). J Crano-Maxillofac Surg 24 [Suppl 1]:133
18. Ewers R, Härle F (1985) Experimental and clinical results of new advances in the treatment of facial trauma. Plastic Reconstr Surg 75:25–31
19. Gay B, Bucher H (1985) Tierexperimentelle Untersuchungen zur Anwendung von absorbierbaren Osteosyntheseschrauben aus Polydioxanon (PDS). Unfallchirurg 88:126–133
20. Gluck T (1888) Referat über die durch das moderne chirurgische Experiment gewonnenen positiven Resultate. Langenbecks Arch 41: 187–239; 747–748
21. Heine C (1878) Über operative Behandlung der Pseudarthrosen. Arch Klin Chir 22:472–495
22. Herold A, Bruch H, Weckbach A, Romen W, Schönefeld G (1988) Polyhydroxybuttersäure – ein biodegenerables Osteosynthesematerial? Hefte zur Unfallheilkunde, Heft 200, Springer, Berlin Heidelberg New York, S665–666
23. Hoffmann G, Kreitek C, Haas N, Tscherne H (1989) Die distale Radiusfraktur. Frakturstabilisierung mit biodegradierbaren Osteosynthese-Stiften (Biofix®). Experimentelle Untersuchungen und erste klinische Erfahrungen. Unfallchirurg 92:430–434
24. Kawaguchi T, Nakano M, Juni K, Inoue S (1983) Examination of biodegradability of poly(ethylene carbonate) and poly(propylene carbonate) in the peritoneal cavity in rats. Chem Pharm Bull 31:1400–1403
25. Kleine J, Kleine H (1959) Über hochmolekulare, insbesondere optisch aktive Polyester der Milchsäure. Ein Beitrag zur Stereochemie makromolekularer Verbindungen. Makromol Chem 30:23–38
26. Knoop M, Lünstedt B, Thiede A (1987) Maxon und PDS – Bewertung physikalischer und biologischer Eigenschaften monofiler, absorbierbarer Nahtmaterialien. Langenbecks Arch Chir 371:13–28
27. Kohn J, Langer R (1986) Poly(iminocarbonates) as potential biomaterials. Biomaterials 7:176–182
28. Kronenthal R (1975) Biodegradable polymers in medicine and surgery. In: Kronenthal R, Oser Z, Martin E (eds) Polymers in medicine and surgery. Plenum Press, New York London, pp119–137
29. Kunz E (1995) Resorbierbare Kunststoffe: Experimentelle Studien über drei Anwendungsbereiche in der Chirurgie. Habilitationsschrift, Universität Würzburg
30. Leong K, Brott B, Langer R (1985) Bioerodible polyanhydrides as drug-carrier matrices. I. Characterization, degradation and release characteristics. J Biomed Mater Res 19:941–955
31. Lister J (1904) Observations on ligature of arteries on the antiseptic system. Lancet I: 451
32. Lowe CE (1954) U.S. Pat. No 2 668 162
33. Maguire J, Coscia M, Lynch M (1987) Foreign body reaction to polymeric debris following total hip arthroplasty. Clin Orthop 216:213–223
34. Merwald M (1995) Resorptionsverhalten und Biokompatibilität von sechs verschiedenen Hydroxycarbonsäuren im Muskelgewebe. Thesis, Universität Würzburg
35. Niederdellmann H, Bührmann K (1983) Vorläufige Mitteilung. Resorbierbare Osteosyntheseschrauben aus Polydioxanon (PDS). Dtsch Z Mund Kiefer Gesichts Chir 7:399–400
36. Pistner H (1992) Osteosynthese mit Blinddübeln und Platten aus biodegradierbarem Block-Poly-(L-Lactid). Akademischer Verlag, München
37. Pistner H (1999) Osteosynthese mit resorbierbaren Materialien. Einhorn-Presse, Reinbek
38. Pistner H, Gutwald R, Mühling J (1991) Biodegradation von resorbierbaren Osteosynthesematerialien. Biomed Tech 36 [Suppl]:114–115
39. Pistner H, Gutwald R, Ordung O, Mühling J, Reuther J (1993a) Poly(l-lactide): a long-term degradation study in vivo. I. Biological results. Biomaterials 14:671–677
40. Pistner H, Bendix D, Mühling J, Reuther J (1993b) Poly(l-lactide): a long-term degradation study in vivo. Part III. Analytical characterization. Biomaterials 14:291–298

41. Pistner H, Stallforth H, Gutwald R, Mühling J, Reuther J (1994) Poly(l-lactide): a long-term degradation study in vivo. Part II: Physico-mechanical behaviour of implants. Biomaterials 15:439–450
42. Pistner H, Reuther J, Kübler N, Bill J (1995) Perspektiven biodegradierbarer Materialien. Biomed Tech 40 [Suppl 3]:24–27
43. Pitt C, Jeffcoat A, Zweidinger R, Schindler (1979) Sustained drug delivery systems. I. The permeability of poly(ε-caprolactone), poly (D,L-lactid acid) and their copolymers. J Biomed Mater Res 13:497–507
44. Pitt C, Gratzl M, Kimmel G, Surles J, Schindler A (1981) Aliphatic polyesters II. The degradation of poly(D,L-lactide), poly(ε-caprolactone) and their copolymers in vivo. Biomaterials 2:215–220
45. Ray J, Doddi N, Regula D, Williams J, Melveger A (1981) Poydioxanone (PDS), a novel monofilament synthetic absorbable suture. Surg Gynecol Obstet 153:497–507
46. Richards M, Dahiyat B, Arm D, Brown P, Leong K (1991) Evaluation of polyphosphates and polyphosphonates as degradable biomaterials. J Biomed Mat Res 25:1151–1167
47. Roby M, Casey D, Cody R (1985) Absorbable sutures based on glycolide/trimethylene carbonate copolymers. Trans Soc Biomater 8:216
48. Roed-Petersen, B (1974) Absorbable Synthetic Suture Material for Internal Fixation of Fractures of the Mandible. Int J Oral Surg 3:133–136
49. Rokkanen P, Böstman O, Vainionpää S, Vihtonen K, Törmälä P, Laihio J, Kilpikari J (1985) Biodegradable implants in fracture fixation: early results in treatment of fractures of the ankle. Lancet I:1422–1424
50. Scheele C (1780) Om Mjölk, och dess Syra. Kgl. Vetenskaps-Academiens nya Handlingar (Stockholm) 1:116–124
51. Schlosshauer B, Steuer H, Müller E, Planck H (2002) Entwicklungen für eine resorbierbare Nervenleitschiene. Biomaterialien 3:191–196
52. Schmitt E (1967) Surgical sutures. US Patent 3297033
53. Shalaby S u. Jamiolkowski D (1985) Absorbable fibres of ε-caprolactone/glycolide copolymers and their biological properties. Polm Prepr 26:200
54. Socin (1887) cited according to Illi (1992) Correspondenzblatt für Schweizer Aerzte 12:11
55. Susruta cited according to Nockemann P (1980) Die chirurgische Naht. Thieme, Stuttgart New York, S1
56. Tsuruta T, Matsuura K, Inoue S (1964) Preparation of some polyesters by organometallic-catalyzed ring opening polymerization. Makromol Chem 75:211–214
57. Woodward S, Brewer P, Moatamed F, Schindler A, Pitt C (1985) The intracellular degradation of poly(ε-caprolactone). J Biomed Mater Res 19:437–444
58. Wüstner M, Partecke B, Buck-Gramcko D (1986) Resorbierbare PDS-Splinte zur Frakturstabilisierung und für Arthrodesen an der Hand. Handchirurgie 18:298–301
59. Youmes H, Nataf P, Cohn D, Appelbaum Y, Pizov G, Uretzky G (1988) Biodegradable PELA block copolymers: in vitro degradation and tissue reaction. Biomat Art Cell Art Org 16:705–719

CHAPTER 12

Photo-oxidized Osteochondral Transplants*   12

BRIGITTE VON RECHENBERG and JÖRG A. AUER

Introduction

The use of osteochondral transplants (OCT) has gained popularity in clinical orthopaedics, mainly as a form of therapy for chronic focal cartilage lesions. In these cases, autografts [19] or allografts [3, 20] are applied either as single plugs, or as mosaicplasty, and multiple osteochondral transplants can be introduced arthroscopically [8, 11]. Most cases are located at the femoral condyle of the knee and less frequently at the talus. Clinical follow-ups revealed a good clinical outcome, however, problems relating to the use of auto- and allografts must be evaluated. Donor site morbidity [1] and repair with fibrocartilaginous tissue were reported using autografts [9, 10]. Aspects of immunology require pretreatment of allografts to avoid graft rejection in addition to the danger of disease transmission [5, 21, 22]. Long-term degeneration of repaired cartilage [10], problems of joint congruency [19], the fusion of graft and host cartilage [2], as well as availability of osteochondral transplants in autografting, stimulated the search for suitable cartilage substitutes. An osteochondral transplant as an "off-the-shelf product" would be ideal. Such a transplant should be readily available, biocompatible, allowing cryoconservation, and withstanding the mechanical load immediately after weight-bearing with primary mechanical stability in the host bed. Photo-oxidized osteochondral xenografts were reported to fulfill some of these requirements. In a long-term experimental study over 18 months in the sheep the fusion of the graft-host cartilaginous interface could be achieved [2, 3].

Process of Photo-Oxidation

Photo-oxidation is a dye mediated process, where after an extensive cleansing procedure the tissue is immersed in a constantly stirred solution of 0.01% methylene blue and exposed to a halogen light source [12] (patent # EP 0768332A1, US 5,817,153).

* Those studies pertaining to photo-oxidized osteochondral grafts were funded by Centerpulse Biologics, Winterthur, Switzerland. The technical and scientific support of Daniel Nadler and Dr. Pedro Bittmann is gratefully acknowledged, as well as the PhD work of Dr. Margarete Akens.

This process alters the configuration of the sulfur bonds and aromatic amino acids, specifically within collagen fibers.

It results in an improved cross-linking of the collagen fibers and thus, better resistance to enzymatic degradation. Apart from affecting mechanical features the process was shown to reduce immunogenic properties [2, 4, 12]. After photo-oxidation, there are no viable chondrocytes left in the cartilage matrix, as proven with live and dead staining (LIVE/DEAD®, Viability/Cytotoxicity Kit; Molecular probes Inc., Jura supply, Switzerland) [3]. Although extensive washing procedures are applied after photo-oxidation. The blue color is retained by the tissue and is clearly visible in the photo-oxidized osteochondral transplants.

Principle of Tissue Guided Regeneration with Photo-Oxidized Osteochondral Transplants

Over time, bone grafts and substitutes are completely replaced with new host bone according to the principle of "creeping substitution" [13]. The bone grafts or substitutes are primarily resorbed, replaced with new woven bone, and finally bone remodeling results in normal lamellar bone, at least in long bones. In contrast to bone grafts, the fate of cartilage or osteochondral grafts is unknown, also for autografts, except that a long-term degeneration of the graft cartilage is also observed [9, 10]. The question, whether these grafts are incorporated or replaced has not been determined. In experimental studies with photo-oxidized xenografts of bovine origin, in the stifle joints of the sheep [2, 3, 16–18] (animals n = 113, grafts n >226), it has been demonstrated that the implanted photo-oxidized osteochondral transplant is substituted by creeping substitution over an 18-month period of both, the bony and the cartilaginous part of the transplant. This was true in single plugs, as well as in mosaicplasty, but unrelated to the structure of the grafts, and was already indicated macroscopically by the disappearance of the bluish color of the original graft (Fig. 12.1).

Remodeling of the bony part was well advanced at 2 months and was generally completed at 6 and/or 12 months. Apart from other influences, the speed of bone remodeling was mainly dependent upon the structure or design of the graft. Mushroom structured grafts were faster remodeled when compared to cylindrical grafts [18]. Remodeling of the calcified cartilage zone and tidemark with cells derived from the subchondral bone area was observed as early as 2 months, and in mushroom structured grafts this process was normally completed within 6 months, if grafts were mechanically stable. In cylindrical grafts, this process took longer but was largely complete at 12 months after implantation. The cells from the subchondral bone area penetrated the calcified cartilage zone, including the tidemark, and started to repopulate the old photo-oxidized cartilage matrix already at 2 months. At 12 months, repopulation of the old matrix with chondrocyte-like cells was normally complete and new matrix synthesis was observed by increased metachromatic staining of the extracellular matrix. Increased pericellular staining distinguished living cells very easily already at 2 months.

Apart from repopulation of the old photo-oxidized matrix from the subchondral bone area some other interesting features were observed with photo-oxidized osteochondral transplants. Matrix flow from the host cartilage towards the graft was always observed, and at 6 months some fusion between the graft and the host cartilage was

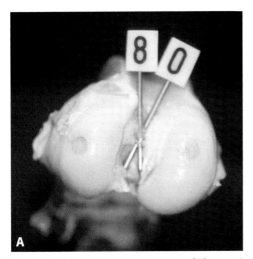

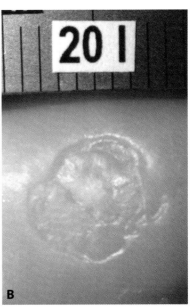

Fig. 12.1A,B. Macroscopic appearance of photo-oxidized cylindrical plugs 6 (**A**) and 18 (**B**) months after surgery. Note that the bluish color of the graft is visible at 6 but not at 18 months.

present, if grafts were mechanically stable. In addition, a small pannus-like tissue covered the graft cartilage from where cells invaded the superficial zone of the graft cartilage (Fig. 12.2). Here clusters and chondrons were detected, as well as increased periterritorial matrix staining. At 18 months, cartilage with a hyaline structure and no signs of cartilage degeneration could be demonstrated with photo-oxidized single cylindrical plugs, whereas in the mosaicplasties with mushroom structured grafts the peripheral but not the central grafts were remodeled already at 12 months. As in bone grafts or substitutes, the "creeping substitution" occurred from the periphery and slowly moved towards the center of the grafts, which in case of the cartilage was the middle zone of the cartilaginous part of the grafts. The original grafts merely served as a three-dimensional scaffold for cells to grow in from the subchondral bone area and pannus covering the surface of the grafts. It was concluded that at least in the cylindrical and mushroom-structured photo-oxidized grafts repair and regeneration of the hyaline cartilage followed the principles of tissue-guided regeneration.

Host-to-Graft Cartilage Interface

Fusion occurring at the host-to-graft or graft-to-graft interface was dependent on several factors. Among those, mechanical stability of the grafts and equal heights at the level of the calcified cartilage zone, including the tidemark [16–18], was important for fusion to occur. Furthermore, cartilage viability in the host cartilage was a pre-requisite that graft and host cartilage could unite (Fig. 12.3A). This was also true for graft-graft-junctions that only occurred if repopulation of matrices had occurred on both sides in mosaicplasty with mushroom-structured grafts. Cluster formation, cell division and

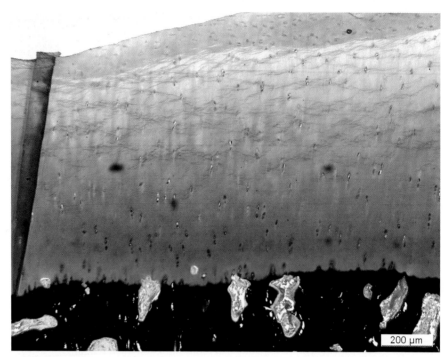

Fig. 12.2. Repopulation of a mushroom structured graft at 6 months. Remodeling of the calcified cartilage zone including the tidemark is visible. Repopulation of the photo-oxidized cartilage matrix is occurring at the superficial and deep cartilage zone as well as new matrix synthesis, indicated by increased metachromatic staining of the extracellular cartilage matrix (ground section, 30–40 μm, surface staining with toluidine blue).

normal metachromatic matrix staining within the host cartilage was seen at 2, 6, 12, and 18 months, with the photo-oxidized cylindrical and mushroom-structured grafts, sometimes even in cases where the grafts had slightly sunk into the original defect. Even then, fusion between the graft and host cartilage could be demonstrated, although in some of these cases the host matrix had grown over the graft matrix (Fig. 12.3B). Experiments conducted with untreated, fresh autogeneic grafts revealed different and much less convincing results. Apart from the fact that matrix staining and repopulation with living chondrocytes was considerably decreased, compared to the photo-oxidized xenografts, the adjacent host cartilage matrix always had a small seam where signs of severe cartilage degeneration were present. Cluster formation and normal matrix staining had already diminished at 6 months after surgery. The reason for the difference of cartilage viability seems to be connected to the pretreatment of the grafts with photo-oxidation, and as a result of this chemical substances, which inhibit matrix degradation, diffuse into the adjacent host cartilage matrix, as indicated by biological markers of cartilage degradation and synthesis [14, 15]. *In vitro* studies with photo-oxidized cartilage showed that incubation of normal bovine cartilage in combination with photo-oxidized cartilage inhibited the activity of neutral metalloproteinases [4].

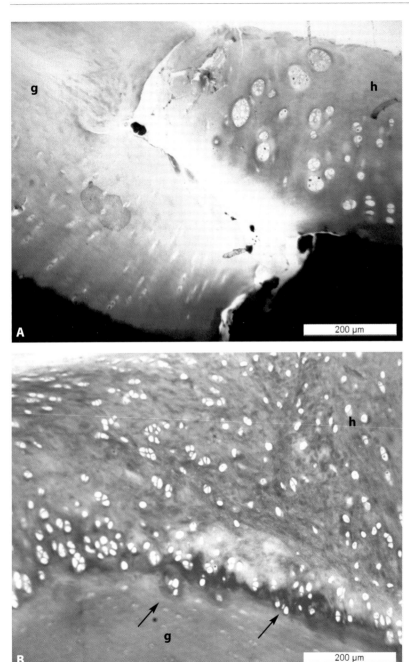

Fig. 12.3A,B. Fusion of the host and graft at the interface in the mushroom structured graft at 6 (**A**) and 12 (**B**) months. The graft matrix (*g*) is not repopulated yet, but viable cells from the host cartilage (*h*) are intruding into the old photo-oxidized graft matrix (*arrows;* 5 µm section, staining with toluidine blue).

Influence of Graft Structure for Graft Survival

In clinical cases of mosaicplasty cylindrical osteochondral grafts are usually applied. Special instruments have been developed for this technique [7] in order to achieve a perfect press-fit between the grafts and the host bed. The problem with using cylindrical grafts is the central necrosis of the mosaicplasty. As with single cylindrical fresh auto- and pretreated allografts [2, 16], this central necrosis is mostly due to a fast resorption of the bony part of the grafts and the temporary replacement with fibrous tissue. The development of cyst-like lesions is the result and can be visualized with diagnostic imaging of clinical patients. However, if collapsing of the graft can be prevented, the cyst-like lesions may resolve and the fibrous tissue finally replaced with bone. If overlapping cylindrical plugs are used, there is the danger of an increase in central necrosis, when compared to where a small seam of host bone is left between the grafts [7, 17]. In our experimental studies it has been shown that cyst formation in the cylindrical grafts always occurred at the base of the grafts or at the graft-host interface. The pathologic bone resorption and the replacement with fibrous tissue at the base of the grafts was thought to be an effect of the mechanical load exerted on the cylindrical grafts, while at the host-graft interface it was mainly attributed to penetration and pressure of synovial fluid during ambulating. Therefore, a new graft design was applied. A mushroom-structured graft was created where the mushroom head ($\varnothing$ 6 mm) consisted of the cartilaginous part, the calcified cartilage zone, including the tidemark and 1 mm of subchondral bone, while the stem was thinner ($\varnothing$ 2.5 mm) and formed only by bone. With this special structure the mechanical load was distributed on two levels, with the larger contact area being at the relatively compact subchondral bone directly underneath the cartilage, and the smaller area of the stem at the level of the more porous and therefore weaker area of the trabecular bone. The overall length of the graft was 8 mm and the stem was strong enough to anchor the grafts securely within the host bone.

Apart from the better mechanical load distribution this mushroom-structure also proved beneficial for other aspects, such as repopulation of the old photo-oxidized cartilage matrix with living cells and the prevention of central necrosis, especially in mosaicplasty. Repopulation was facilitated and enhanced through faster and better accessibility of the calcified cartilage zone by cells from the subchondral bone area [18]. Central necrosis could be better avoided also with overlapping grafts, since more viable host bone was left between the relatively thin stems of the mushroom-structured grafts. This also allowed for better joint congruency. Grafts could be tilted at a slight angle and still have some host bone left between them [17]. Last but not least, the mushroom structure seemed to inhibit efficiently the pumping action of synovial fluid during ambulation and thus preventing cyst formation at the host-graft interface.

Clinical Use: Advantages and Disadvantages

Photo-oxidized osteochondral transplants fulfill several criteria warranted in an "off-the-shelf" product for clinical use in cartilage resurfacing. Major advantages are certainly the availability of these transplants in addition to the prevention of donor site morbidity in clinical patients. As the immunological response to photo-oxidized transplants was reduced, this is an advantage over the allografts already used in clinical orthopaedics. Further to the ease of the surgical application of photo-oxidized transplants it was also found that a mushroom-shaped graft has several advantages over a cylindrical-shaped graft. This was especially true for the speed of graft remodeling. The mushroom structure is only applicable in pretreated grafts, where special equipment is used in preparation under sterile conditions well in advance of the surgical procedure. This could not be performed with autografts, which are harvested during surgery in clinical patients. Therefore, if mushroom-structured grafts should be applied, autografts can not be considered.

Photo-oxidized osteochondral transplants are non-viable transplants, which makes them quite different to most of the currently clinically applied cartilage replacements. Generally, lack of chondrocyte viability is a major concern in the medical literature dealing with cartilage resurfacing. The non-viable cartilage of the photo-oxidized grafts, however, did not seem to be disadvantageous for graft survival. In contrast, the photo-oxidized grafts showed significantly better long-term results in comparison to fresh autografts, where cartilage degeneration was severe at 18 months [2]. It could be speculated that living cells might add to the cartilage degeneration of the grafts through the synthesis and release of matrix metalloproteinases. While in the photo-oxidized cylindrical and mushroom structured grafts new matrix synthesis could be recorded already at 6 and 12 months, this was never observed in the autografts. In addition, the non-viable cartilage and bone matrix of the photo-oxidized grafts may also decrease the immunogenic response in the host tissue.

The disadvantages of photo-oxidized osteochondral grafts may be the use of allo- or xenografts and its related disease transmission. Studies, where the survival of infectious agents (virus etc.) during the manufacturing process will be investigated may be required in the future. However, it may be safe to assume that the process of photo-oxidation may not only kill infectious agents but also alter other protein configurations.

Conclusion

In conclusion, the use of photo-oxidized osteochondral transplants may be a good solution for cartilage resurfacing if focal cartilage defects are present. It may however not be a final solution in avoiding joint replacement. However, the use of photo-oxidized osteochondral transplants may postpone clinical application of the artificial joint replacement for a couple of years and thus improve life quality of human patients considerably.

References

1. Ahmad CS, Guiney WB, Drinkwater CJ (2002) Evaluation of donor site intrinsic healing response in autologous osteochondral grafting of the knee. Arthroscopy 18:95–98
2. Akens MA, Rechenberg Bv, Bittmann P, Nadler D, Zlinszky K, Auer JA (2001) Long term in vivo studies of a photooxidized bovine osteochondral transplant in sheep. BMC Musculoskeletal Disorders 2:1471–2474
3. Akens MK (2002) In-vitro and in-vivo study of osteochondral transplants pretreated with photo-oxidation. PhD thesis, University of Zurich

4. Akens MK, Rechenberg Bv, Bittmann P, Nadler D, Zlinszky K, Auer JA (2002) In vitro studies of a photo-oxidized bovine articular cartilage. J Vet Med A 49:39–45
5. Friedlaender GE, Strong DM, Tomford WW, Mankin HJ (1999) Long-term follow-up of patients with osteochondral allografts. A correlation between immunologic responses and clinical outcome. Orthop Clin North Am 30:583–588
6. Garrett JC (1994) Fresh osteochondral allografts for treatment of articular defects in osteochondritis dissecans of the lateral femoral condyle in adults. Clin Orthop 303:33–37
7. Hangody L, Kish G (1996) Smith & Nephew Endoscopy. MosaicPlastyTM Osteochondral Grafting
8. Hangody L, Kish G, Karpati Z, Szerb I, Udvarhelyi I (1997) Arthroscopic autogenous osteochondral mosaicplasty for the treatment of femoral condylar articular defects. A preliminary report. Knee Surg Sports Traumatol Arthrosc 5:262–267
9. Hunziker EB (1999) Articular cartilage repair: are the intrinsic biological constraints undermining this process insuperable? Osteoarthritis Cartilage 7:15–28
10. Hunziker EB, Rosenberg L (1997) Articular cartilage repair. In: Koopman WJ (ed) Arthritis and allied conditions, 13th edn, vol 2. Williams &Wilkins, Baltimore, pp2027–2038
11. Matsusue Y, Yamamuro T, Hama H (1993) Arthroscopic multiple osteochondral transplantation to the chondral defect in the knee associated with anterior cruciate ligament disruption. Arthroscopy 9:318–321
12. Moore M, Bohachewski I, Cheung D et al. (1994) Stabilization of pericardial tissue by dye mediated photooxidation. J Biomed Mater Res 28:611–618
13. Phemister D (1914) The fate of transplanted bone and regenerative power of various constituents. Surg Gynecol Obstet 19:303–333
14. Poole AR (2000) Cartilage in health and disease. In: McCarty DJ, Koopman WJ (eds) Arthritis and allied conditions, 13th edn, vol 1. Lea & Febiger, Philadelphia London
15. Poole RA, Paul D (1994) Biological markers in rheumatoid arthritis. Sem Arthritis Rheum 23:17–31
16. Rechenberg B von, Akens MK, Nadler D et al. (2002) Changes in subchondral bone in cartilage resurfacing – an experimental study in sheep using different types of osteochondral grafts (accepted)
17. Rechenberg B von, Akens MK, Nadler D et al. (2003) Mosaicplasty: a comparison between photooxidized mushroom structured and cylindrical grafts in an experimental study with sheep (in preparation)
18. Rechenberg B von, Akens MK, Nadler D et al. (2003) The use of photooxidized, mushroom structured osteochondral grafts for cartilage resurfacing – a comparison to photooxidized cylindrical grafts in an experimental study in sheep (submitted)
19. Sanders TG, Mentzer KD, Miller MD, Morrison WB, Campbell SE, Penrod BJ (2001) Autogenous osteochondral "plug" transfer for the treatment of focal chondral defects: postoperative MR appearance with clinical correlation. Skeletal Radiol 30:570–578
20. Schachar NS, Novak K, Hurtig M et al. (1999) Transplantation of cryopreserved osteochondral dowel allografts for repair of focal articular defects in an ovine model. J Orthop Res 17:909–920
21. Stevenson SS, Dannucci GA, Sharkey NA, Pool RR (1989) The fate of articular cartilage after transplantation of fresh and cryopreserved tissue-antigen-matched and mismatched osteochondral allografts in dogs. J Bone Joint Surg-A 71:1297–1307
22. Strong DM, Friedlaender GE, Tomford WW et al. (1996) immunological responses in human recipients of osseous and osteochondral grafts. Clin Orthop 326:107–114

Cells for Cartilage Repair

V

CHAPTER 13

Chondrocytes 13

ACHIM BATTMANN, THOMAS NUSSELT, LARS WALZ, MARKUS SCHALLER, CHRISTIAN HENDRICH, LUDGER FINK, HOLGER HAAS, INGKE JÜRGENSEN and ULRICH STAHL

Introduction

A chondrocyte is a cell producing or maintaining a surrounding matrix.

However, it has to be recognized that there is a whole group of cells named "chondrocytes", which fulfill a completely different set of functions (Fig. 13.1).

The most commonly recognized chondrocyte is the chondrocyte found in the articular cartilage, which will be the major point of discussion in this paper. Other types of condrocytes are found in the meniscus (e.g. of the knee) maintaining a fibrous cartilage, and within the intervertebral disc. Also, chondrocytes are found during bone development and bone repair. In early bone formation, chondrocytes are found in growth areas of long bones, a process known as enchondral ossification. After the end

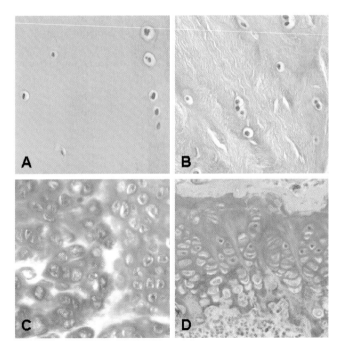

Fig. 13.1A–D. Different types of chondrocytes (all pictures alcian blue staining, 400×). (A) Hyaline cartilage, (B) meniscus. (C) callus tissue, (D) growth plate of juvenile bone.

of skeletal growth, chondrocytes can be found after fracture during bone repair in the callus tissue. Therefore, the term chondrocyte is used for a variety of cells having different functions (see Fig. 13.1) [11].

Development

The chondrocyte follows a defined way of differentiation. From the stem cell it changes to an "early" chondroblast. The major property of which is mitotic reproduction to create a sufficient number of cells for the generation of an appropriate amount of cartilage matrix. At this time, the developing chondrocyte is called a "proliferating chondroblast". After enough cells have been generated the proliferating chondroblast changes into a "producing chondroblast". This cell type generates the matrix of the joint surfaces. Finally, the chondroblast becomes a differentiated chondrocyte with its typical bi-cellular appearance.

Matrix

Articular chondrocytes are embedded in an extracellular matrix, which is predominantly composed of collagen type II, proteoglycans, and water. These components are arranged in a sophisticated network, which provides the unique elasticity and rigidity necessary for articular cartilage. The matrix is found in the vicinity of the chondrocyte in 2 forms, as a territorial and an interterritorial matrix. The territorial matrix is only a very small portion of the matrix and can be seen as a halo around the chondrocytes. It contains matrix components, which have not been formed into the typical three-dimensional structure [11]. The interterritorial matrix is the major component of the articular cartilage and contains the interconnected collagens and proteoglycans, binding the water molecules. This matrix is the final product of the articular chondrocytes. The half-life of the matrix is estimated about 100 years (Fig. 13.2) [1].

Nucleus

Territorial Matrix

Interterritorial Matrix

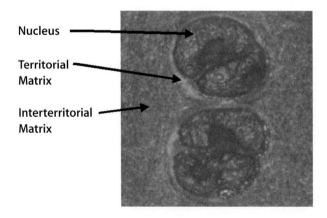

Fig. 13.2.
Typical chondrocyte in hyaline cartilage with bi-cellular appearance and territorial and interterritorial matrix area. Laser scanning microscopy, 1000×.

Nutrition

Chondrocyte nutrition is provided by the anaerobic glycogen metabolism of the synovial fluid [15]. This is unique, because almost all other cells in the body depend on oxygen metabolism. Furthermore, compared to blood, only a selected pool of growth factors is supplied. The nutrition is maintained by diffusion. Therefore, the thickness of the cartilage is dependent on the distance that energy carriers can cover. Thus, the thickness of the articular cartilage layer is evolutionary limited.

In contrast, the bone forming (enchondral) chondrocytes are nurtured by blood. The cells have an oxidative metabolism and are exposed to a wide spectrum of growth factors and hormones. However, the function of these chondrocytes is completely different. Once bone formation is finished the cells vanish completely. While articular chondrocytes with their slow anaerobic metabolism are obviously made for lifetime, bone forming chondrocyte appear only during skeletal growth and are replaced by bone tissue. Only during bone remodeling after fractures these chondrocytes appear again for a limited time in callus tissue. *In vitro* experiments have proven the effect of oxygen concentration on chondrocytes leading to high matrix production at higher concentrations and vice versa [17]. This fact has important implications for tissue regeneration.

Degeneration and Regeneration

Degeneration

Degeneration is mainly observed in articular cartilage and is known as osteoarthritis. The most important risk factors are overweight and age [16]. Thus, articular cartilage seems to be especially prone to "wear and tear" since regenerative processes as found in other parenchymal organs such as the liver are not existing. This hypothesis is further supported by the fact that disturbances in the normal joint function accelerates osteoarthritis. Osteoarthritis after meniscectomy in the knee joint can be used as an example. Normally, the intact meniscus regulates the distribution of weight through the whole articular surface. After removing parts of the meniscus, other parts of the joint are exposed to an increased load, which results in higher compression of the cartilage matrix. This leads to a hardening of the matrix and an impaired diffusion of nutrients and finally to a disturbed chondrocyte function. As a consequence, the matrix can not be maintained and gets destroyed by mechanical stress, visible as fibrillations and separation of the cartilage surface [14]. One reaction of the chondrocytes close to these areas is the formation of cell clusters, typically seen in osteoarthritic cartilage. However, it is known that cartilage does not heal and the cluster formation must be seen as an indicator and failed attempt of repair. As already pointed out earlier the articular chondrocyte seems to be a lifetime cell. This is also supported by the immense half-life of the matrix, exceeding the normal human life expectancy. Obviously, a regeneration of the articular matrix from a stem cell pool as seen in many other organs is physiologically not intended. In contrast, in callus tissue, typical cartilage cells can be found. This fact suggests that at least in the bone there are still inducible stem cells present.

For the differentiation of articular cartilage cells the lack of an oxidative cell metabolism seems to be mandatory. All studies working on articular cartilage repair (e.g. the autologous chondrocyte transplantation) and matrix-based cell transplantation systems stress the extreme importance of a completely blood free transplantation site. Obviously, the presence of an anaerobic metabolism seems to be of major importance for the maintenance of the chondrogenic phenotype.

Regeneration

Regeneration of articular cartilage tissue "ad integrum" is not occurring. Initially, defects are filled by a fibrous scar tissue, a form of defect healing as seen elsewhere in the body. Finally a "fibrocartilaginous" tissue can be found, which is a mixture of a fibrous scar and a tissue with cartilaginous properties, e.g. the expression of cartilage-specific collagen type II and other collagens [24]. Looking at morphological criteria, even the most advanced methods of tissue engineering and cartilage repair still fail to produce the typical phenotype of hyaline cartilage.

Chondrocytes in Vitro

Chondrocytes grown *in vitro* is one of the most important techniques for cartilage repair today. The cultivation of *in vitro* cartilage cells has been pioneered already more than 20 years ago, and was consequently used for the autologous chondrocyte transplantation method by Peterson [19]. Initially, cells were grown using standard monolayer *in vitro* systems. Growing the cells in three-dimensional clusters using carries like alginate or collagens is more appropriate [12, 22].

Cartilage cells grown *in vitro* can not be identified by morphological methods. Their differentiation is determined by the detection of cartilage-specific proteins like collagen types II, IX, and XI. A loss of differentiation can be determined by the production of collagen types I, III, and X. The products can be identified either on the protein level by specific assays or by immunohistochemical staining. The detection can also be performed on the mRNA level by quantitative reverse transcription polymerase chain reaction (qRT-PCR). This method allows the measurement of additional factors not directly connected with secreted products including the transcription factor Cbfa-1 (osf-2, runx-2), a member of the runt superfamily of transcription factors. Cbfa-1 was first discovered as an early differentiation factor of the osteoblastic lineage. Later its presence could be detected also in cartilage cells.

Differentiation, De-Differentiation and Plasticity

As pointed out earlier, there are certain proteins, which are specific for differentiated chondrocytes, as well as others for de-differentiated chondrocytes. The term "de-differentiation" suggests that a cell differentiates backwards to a less committed stage of differentiation. Is that a plausible hypothesis? When looking at other tissues in the body there is a programmed repair mechanism initiated from local stem cells. However, why should a differentiated cell return to a stem cell level? As stressed earlier, there is no stem cell compartment in the articular cartilage. Thus, the attempts of tissue repair must be generated by the cartilage cells themselves.

A more likely hypothesis is therefore the concept of plasticity. This means that the cells do not regress to a previous level of differentiation, but merely switch their differentiation into another phenotype. Cells connected to the chondrogenic phenotype are osteoblasts and fibroblasts, as can be demonstrated by enchondral ossification and the formation of cartilaginous callus tissue after bone fracture.

We could demonstrate the plasticity of chondrocytes by the expression of the differentiation marker cbfa1 *in vitro*. Cbfa-1 is a transcription factor initially thought to be an essential and exclusive pre-requisite for osteogenic differentiation [6]. However, its presence in chondrocytes became acknowledged and is of increasing interest [13, 23]. Freshly isolated human articular chondrocytes showed a basal expression of Cbfa-1. Continuously grown in monolayer cultures they present an increasing expression of this differentiation factor, up to 215% of its initial value. Returned into a three-dimensional alginate culture system the expression of Cbfa-1 drops close to the detection level. After an extended time period it is only slightly increasing (Fig. 13.3). These results suggest two important conclusions. First, the articular chondrocytes do not de-differentiate in monolayer cultures *in vitro*, but switch into another more osteoblastic phenotype. Once put in a three-dimensional culture system they differentiate again into a chondrogenic phenotype, indicating a typical plastically behavior (Fig. 13.4) [3, 7, 9]. Secondly, the three-dimensional structure of the cell environment seems to be an essential pre-requisite for the maintenance of the chondrogenic phenotype [4, 8, 21].

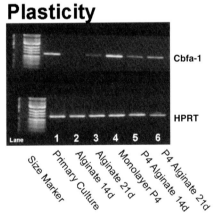

Fig. 13.3. Plasticity of chondrocytes. Influence of monolayer and three-dimensional culture conditions on Cbfa-1 expression in human articular chondrocytes. High expression of Cbfa-1 in monolayer cultures during the first and fourth passage (lane 1 and 4). Decreased expression in a three-dimensional alginate system in primary chondrocytes after 2 and 3 weeks (lane 2 and 3), and after 4 passages in monolayer cultures (lane 5 and 6). HPRT was used as a control.

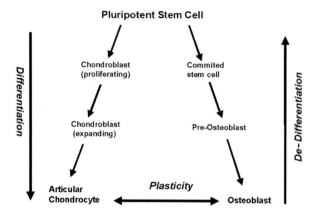

Fig. 13.4.
Illustration of differentiation, de-differentiation and plasticity. Possible cell differentiation in vertical and horizontal directions.

Conclusion

Chondrocytes are found in articular cartilage, in enchondral ossification, in callus tissue, and in fibrocartilage. There is evidence that they can change their differentiation and phenotype. The chondrocyte is not only defined by its individual cellular properties and functions but also by its surrounding tissue, which is in the case of the articular chondrocytes the collagenous matrix. In articular cartilage there is no pool of stem cells. A repair of defects by a recruitment of stem cells as seen in other organs is not possible. Chondrocytes expanded *in vitro* are an attempt to repair articular cartilage defects. The cells can be used in the ACT procedure or seeded onto a carrier matrix. Histomorphologically these systems still fail to produce a typical hyaline-like cartilage. As shown by our results, a matrix-based culture system has advantages compared to monolayer cell cultures. Stem cells for chondrogenic differentiation needed during enchondral ossification and fracture healing are present in bone marrow [20, 26]. These mesenchymal stem cells can be isolated but a way to differentiate them into hyaline-like articular chondrocytes has to be identified. Pre-requisites are the depletion of oxygen to move them into a non-oxidative cell metabolism and the use of a carrier matrix. The engineering of articular cartilage from stem cells has different advantages [18]. A major one is that intact articular cartilage must not be sacrificed. Cartilage repair with stem cells might become available in the near future, resulting in shortening of the healing process, and improvement of joint function [1, 5, 10, 25].

References

1. Aigner T, Kim HA (2002) Apoptosis and cellular vitality: issues in osteoarthritic cartilage degeneration. Arthritis Rheum 46:1986–1996
2. Angele P, Kujat R, Nerlich M, Yoo J, Goldberg V, Johnstone B (1999) Engineering of osteochondral tissue with bone marrow mesenchymal progenitor cells in a derivatized hyaluronan-gelatin composite sponge. Tissue Eng 5:545–554

3. Bahrami S, Stratmann U, Wiesmann HP, Mokrys K, Bruckner P, Szuwart T (2000) Periosteally derived osteoblast-like cells differentiate into chondrocytes in suspension culture in agarose. Anat Rec 259:124–130
4. Chubinskaya S, Huch K, Schulze M, Otten L, Aydelotte MB, Cole AA (2001) Gene expression by human articular chondrocytes cultured in alginate beads. J Histochem Cytochem 49:1211–1220
5. de Crombrugghe B, Lefebvre V, Nakashima K (2001) Regulatory mechanisms in the pathways of cartilage and bone formation. Curr Opin Cell Biol 13:721–727
6. Ducy P, Zhang R, Geoffroy V, Ridall AL, Karsenty G (1997) Osf2/Cbfa1: a transcriptional activator of osteoblast differentiation. Cell 30:747–754
7. Gerstenfeld LC, Cruceta J, Shea CM, Sampath K, Barnes GL, Einhorn TA (2002) Chondrocytes provide morphogenic signals that selectively induce osteogenic differentiation of mesenchymal stem cells. J Bone Miner Res 17:221–230
8. Hauselmann HJ, Fernandes RJ, Mok SS et al. (1994) Phenotypic stability of bovine articular chondrocytes after long-term culture in alginate beads. J Cell Sci 107:17–27
9. Hegert C, Kramer J, Hargus G et al. (2002) Differentiation plasticity of chondrocytes derived from mouse embryonic stem cells. J Cell Sci 115:4617–4628
10. Im GI, Kim DY, Shin JH, Hyun CW, Cho WH (2001) Repair of cartilage defect in the rabbit with cultured mesenchymal stem cells from bone marrow. J Bone Joint Surg-Br 83:289–294
11. Jee WS (1988) Skeletal tissues. In: Weiss L (ed) Cell and tissue biology, 6th edn. Urban & Schwarzenberg, Baltimore, München
12. Jubel A, Andermahr J, Koebke J, Hauselmann HJ, Rehm KE (2002) Treatment of defects of joint cartilage. Dtsch Med Wochenschr 127:1904–1908
13. Kim IS, Otto F, Zabel B, Mundlos S (1999) Regulation of chondrocyte differentiation by Cbfa1. Mech Dev 80:159–170
14. Kurz B, Jin M, Patwari P, Cheng DM, Lark MW, Grodzinsky AJ (2001) Biosynthetic response and mechanical properties of articular cartilage after injurious compression. J Orthop Res 19:1140–1146
15. Lee DA, Salih V, Stockton EF, Stanton JS, Bentley G (1997) Effect of normal synovial fluid on the metabolism of articular chondrocytes in vitro. Clin Orthop 342:228–238
16. Martin JA, Buckwalter JA (2002) Aging, articular cartilage chondrocyte senescence and osteoarthritis. Biogerontology 3:257–264
17. Murphy CL, Sambanis A (2001) Effect of oxygen tension on chondrocyte extracellular matrix accumulation. Connect Tissue Res 42:87–96
18. Perka C, Schultz O, Spitzer RS, Lindenhayn K (2000) The influence of transforming growth factor beta1 on mesenchymal cell repair of full-thickness cartilage defects. J Biomed Mater Res 52:543–552
19. Peterson L, Minas T, Brittberg M, Nilsson A, Sjogren-Jansson E, Lindahl A (2000) Two- to 9-year outcome after autologous chondrocyte transplantation of the knee. Clin Orthop 374:212–234
20. Pittenger MF, Mackay AM, Beck SC et al. (1999) Multilineage potential of adult human mesenchymal stem cells. Science 284:143–147
21. Reiter I, Tzukerman M, Maor G (2002) Spontaneous differentiating primary chondrocytic tissue culture: a model for endochondral ossification. Bone 31:333–339
22. Schulze M, Kuettner KE, Cole AA (2000) Adult human chondrocytes in alginate culture. Preservation of the phenotype for further use in transplantation models. Orthopäde 29:100–106
23. Stricker S, Fundele R, Vortkamp A, Mundlos S (2002) Role of Runx genes in chondrocyte differentiation. Dev Biol 245:95–108
24. Tew S, Redman S, Kwan A et al. (2001) Differences in repair responses between immature and mature cartilage. Clin Orthop 391 [Suppl]:S142–152
25. Wakitani S, Goto T, Pineda SJ, Young RG, Mansour JM, Caplan AI, Goldberg VM (1994) Mesenchymal cell-based repair of large, full-thickness defects of articular cartilage. J Bone Joint Surg-A 76:579–592
26. Yoo JU, Barthel TS, Nishimura K, Solchaga L, Caplan AI, Goldberg VM, Johnstone B (1998) The chondrogenic potential of human bone-marrow-derived mesenchymal progenitor cells. J Bone Joint Surg Am 80:1745–1757

CHAPTER 14

Quality Assurance of Autologous Chondrocyte Transplantation (ACT)* 14

WILHELM K. AICHER, CHRISTOPH GAISSMAIER and JÜRGEN FRITZ

Introduction

New surgical treatment strategies and the success of transplantation techniques increased the demand for tissue and donor organs [12]. Physicians and scientists from different disciplines joined together and developed techniques to treat patients using biocompatible implants, and the self-healing capacity of the injured or diseased tissue. This strategy was successfully applied to heal bone and dermal defects using resorbable mineral scaffolds and textile-aided wound healing sites. However, the healing capacity of hyaline-like cartilage is very limited. Without treatment, minor chondral or osteo-chondral lesions are thought to progress into major articular cartilage defects [15]. Consequently, techniques to treat articular cartilage defects had to be developed [4].

Brittberg and colleagues described a novel method called autologous chondrocytes transplantation (ACT) [3, 4]. The chondrocytes used for the transplantation are taken from articular cartilage at a remote and healthy site of the affected joint. Cells are expanded *in vitro* and reimplanted into the defect. The articular joint is opened by an arthrotomy, the defect is cleaned from debris, covered with a periostal flap, and the chondrocyte suspension is injected into the defect chamber. The advantages of this approach are that the whole process can be carried out with autologous cells and serum compounds, thus minimizing the risk of an infection from heterologous donor tissue or blood. Further, the affected joint itself serves as a cell source, thus avoiding harm to healthy joints. The success of this method inspired many laboratories to develop variations of the original procedure.

As increasing numbers of patients prefer ACT instead of established surgical procedures for biological cartilage repair, e.g. microfracture or mosaicplasty, the health industry developed both, novel surgical instruments and chondrocyte expansion services for ACT. At the same time, the ACT technique begun to spread out from the very few centers, which had originally developed the skills of ACT. As a consequence, the technique became available for the general orthopaedic surgeon. Today, more than 7000 ACT procedures are performed on an annual basis in the Western Hemisphere. More than a million knee surgeries are performed in Europe and North America each year and an estimated number of about 30,000 to 50,000 of these patients could possibly be better treat-

* This work was supported by BMBF grant 031 26 26 A and in part by DFG grants Ai 16/10, Ai-16/14, and institutional funding.

ed with ACT.[1] Such a demand needs quality standards by the medical societies, the administrations, and the health industry [1, 2, 5].

Quality Management and Quality Assurance for Autologous Chondrocyte Transplantation

Quality assurance for ACT affects all levels of the process. This includes the diagnosis, surgical skills, cell culture techniques, and logistics. The patient considered for ACT treatment has to meet the general diagnostic criteria in the affected joint, as listed below. In young patients (up to 18 years) spontaneous cartilage repair was observed and therefore ACT should not be performed. On the other hand, spontaneous repair capabilities decline over time and consequently patients older than 50 years may not be treated successfully [13]. ACT should only be suggested if the defect is a grade III or IV lesion according to the Outerbridge classification [14], and meets the diagnostic inclusion criteria set by the consensus conferences of the surgical societies. A detailed list of diagnostic criteria was published recently and is available via the internet[2].

General Conditions of the Affected Joint to be Considered for ACT Treatment

- A defined, full-thickness cartilage defect with intact rim and otherwise healthy full-thickness cartilage
- Intact corresponding cartilage areas, no kissing lesion
- Mostly intact meniscus
- A maximum of 2 non-corresponding defects
- Intact tendon function and physiological articular angles
- Free articular mobility

Diagnostic Criteria to Consider ACT Treatment According to the Consensus Conferences

A Inclusion criteria
  - Defect size approx. 2.5 to approx. 10 cm^2, full depth defect, but intact subchondral bone plate
  - Knee: defect localization medial/lateral femur condylus, trochlea, patella
  - Ankle: central talus
  - Diagnosis: osteochondritis dissecans
B Exclusion criteria
  - Defect size smaller than 2 cm^2 or exceeding 14 cm^2, deep (>7 mm) osteochondral defects
  - Diagnosis: inflammatory cartilage destruction including rheumatoid arthritis, reactive or infective arthritis and osteoarthritis, arthofibrosis, ankylosis, mal-alignments (patella, articular axis), carbon implant pins/pegs

---

[1] http://www.sportsinjurybulletin.com/archive/1074-cartilage-transplants.htm; http://www.health.state.mn.us/htac/ac.htm.

[2] http://www.thieme.de/zfo/02_02/ortho_16.html

Expanding High Quality Chondrocytes from Cartilage Biopsies

The chondrocytes used for ACT are normally isolated from small biopsies taken from intact and non weight-bearing areas of the affected joint, such as the intercondylar notch of a knee. Special surgical instruments were developed to harvest the full-thickness cartilage by arthroscopy (e.g. arthoscopy instruments, including Trephine). After harvest, the biopsy is sent to a tissue engineering facility meeting the quality requirements set by public health administration.

Isolation, expansion and quality assurance of chondrocytes for ACT are strictly controlled by public authorities, as such chondrocytes represent a "drug non-ready for use". Therefore, a state of the art quality management regimen to guide and control all steps involved with the collection of tissue, preparation of chondrocytes, and implantation was developed recently.

The challenge of chondrocyte expansion is the fact that these cells de-differentiate during expansion from a chondrogenic to a fibroblast-like phenotype (Fig. 14.1). This de-differentiation is accompanied by a decreasing capacity of the cells to generate a hyaline-like cartilage [7]. The de-differentiation process already starts in primary cultures and after 4 to 5 population doublings the de-differentiation results in cells which express high levels of collagen type I (a1 and a2 genes) and low levels of collagen type II (Fig. 14.2). Furthermore, the expression of other genes including activin-like kinase-1 (ALK-1), bone morphogenetic proteins (BMP) -2 and -4, connective tis-

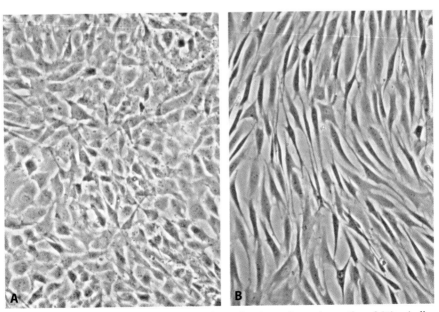

Fig. 14.1A,B. (A) Chondrocytes in primary culture showing polygonal growth and (B) spindle-shaped morphology after numerous passages.

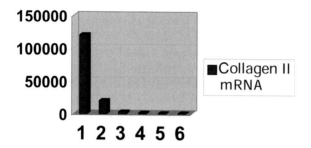

Fig. 14.2.
Levels of mRNA of primary chondrocytes. Collagen type II is high (1) but drops after passaging with each subculture (2–6).

sue growth factor CTGF, growth differentiation factor (GDF) -5, and different interleukins (IL) change during expansion of primary cultured chondrocytes. The elevated levels of IL-1 and IL-18 are associated with an inflammatory situation and elevated expression of such factors is a hallmark of arthritis and a catabolic situation of cartilage. Quality management of chondrocyte expansion for ACT should include the measurement of these factors. Consequently, as a quality standard of the chondrocytes after expansion, and prior to ACT, sufficient expression of collagen type II and aggrecan should be monitored, as well as a low expression of some of the pro-inflammatory factors mentioned above, including IL-1. Besides those phenotypic characteristics an excellent chondrocyte viability and sufficient numbers of cells after expansion are a pre-requisite for a successful ACT.

The cellular quality of the chondrocytes, as outlined above, is just one of the important criteria for ACT. A second pre-requisite is absolute sterility. As cartilage contains no blood or lymph vessels, defense against infections is very poor in this tissue. Furthermore, diffusion of low molecular weight compounds including antibiotics from the synovial tissue and synovial fluid into articular cartilage is also limited. Therefore, all steps in ACT must be performed under strictly sterile conditions. The challenge starts at the arthroscopic surgery. Special instruments for harvesting the cartilage biopsies and for the transportation to the into cell culture facilities were developed (Fig. 14.3).

After isolation of the chondrocytes and during expansion all cell culture equipment and cultures are monitored for possible contamination, including anaerobic and aerobic prokaryotes, mycoplasma, and other microorganisms. Most antibiotics used routinely for cell culture are more bacteriostatic but not bacteriolytic or bactericide. This also applies to agents against mycoplasma or yeast. To avoid low titer contamination of the *in vitro* cultures, that may develop into sepsis after implantation, antibiotics are omitted in all stages of the cell expansion. The final hygiene testing is performed with an aliquot of the cells and the media, just before the materials are transported to the hospital. Incubation and evaluation by microbiological techniques may take a week or more. To ensure the highest safety for the patients, a very sensitive polymerase chain reaction (PCR) may be used to search for most common contaminants including virus, bacteria, mycoplasma, and yeast. A suitable PCR reaction takes less than 1 hour, including analysis of the data. At the same time, a PCR enables the cell culture facilities to prove the phenotypic quality of the chondrocytes after expansion. Therefore, during preparation of the cells for shipment a

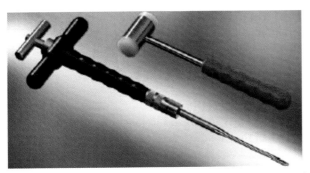

Fig. 14.3. Special designed ACT instruments (developed by Aesculap®, Tuttlingen, Germany) to harvest full-thickness cartilage biopsies. The trephine (*left*) is introduced into the joint under arthroscopical control. The cartilage biopsy (4 mm Ø, 9 mm height) containing the hyaline cartilage, tide mark, and calcified cartilage, is carefully harvested using a hammer (*right*). The depth of the punch can be monitored by a visible scale on the tip of the trephine. By a screw-thread mechanism the cartilage biopsy is pressed out of the trephine into a container with medium to cool and preserve the vital cartilage during transportation.

quality sheet of each batch of chondrocytes is filled out to warrant the quality of the product.

Quality Management by Professional Education

A third component of quality management addresses the education of the people involved in ACT, and the logistics of transportation. Surgeons and health professionals in the hospitals must be trained for optimal harvest and transplantation applicable to ACT. Optimal biopsies contain full-thickness articular cartilage. The biopsy taken, as well as the autologous blood, must be, cooled to 4 °C immediately after collection and during the entire transport to the cell culture facility. However, don't freeze samples at any time, as freeze-thawing cycles, even in the presence of freeze-protective compounds, such as DMSO, drastically reduce the viability of chondrocytes. At the time of surgery, preparation of the cartilage defect and the periostal graft, tight suture of the graft without harming the rim, determination of cell suspension volume needed, and many other considerations need some basic education. Therefore, the health industry, the hospitals, and the responsible societies initiated educational programs to serve these purposes.

Conclusion

Transplantation of chondrocytes by injection of the cells into the defect chamber covered with a periostal graft still represents the state-of-the-art treatment for all patients meeting the ACT inclusion criteria [1, 2, 5]. The disadvantages of the classical cell-suspension ACT include that this technique clearly generates a hyper-cellular hyaline-like cartilage and the distribution of cells immediately after injection may not be optimal [17]. Furthermore, in some studies, a zonal heterogeneity and the generation of fibrous tissue were reported in the repair tissue 12 months after ACT [16]. Interestingly, recent studies showed that this classical technique is unsurpassed for its high chances to generate a stable transplant for years [3, 11] and our MRI follow-up studies did not show signs of histological discontinuity of the repair cartilage (unpublished observation).

More recently scaffold-augmented ACT techniques were developed or are in preclinical evaluation [6, 18]. Growth of the chondrocytes on a scaffold would enable the surgeon to apply the implant by arthroscopy thus avoiding the arthrotomy and possibly improving the implant histology at the same time. Although the surgical advantages of scaffold-augmented chondrocyte implantations delivered by an arthoscopical technique can not be neglected, the integration of such scaffolds into the surrounding healthy cartilage, the long-term stability, problems derived from the degradation of the scaffold matrix, including generation of acid or peptide fragments are not satisfactorily solved. Our data suggest that e.g. collagen type I vlies materials may induce expression of pro-inflammatory compounds [9] and others have recently shown that collagen type II fragments induced a stage of hypertrophy in chondrocytes [10]. Clinical evaluation of patients treated with scaffold-augmented chondrocytes showed a weakening of the repair cartilage after 36 months or later [8] indicating that the processes of implant integration into the surrounding tissue and the process of scaffold degradation need further improvement.

References

1. Behrens P et al. (2002) Arbeitsgemeinschaft ACT und Tissue Engineering. DGU Mitteilungen und Nachrichten 45:34
2. Behrens P et al. (2002) Arbeitsgemeinschaft ACT und Tissue Engineering. Z Orthop 140:132–137
3. Bobic V (2000) Autologous chondrocyte transplantation. Am Acad Orthop Surg, Orlando, FL
4. Brittberg M, Lindahl A, Nilsson A, Ohlsson C, Isaksson O, Peterson L (1994) Treatment of deep cartilage defects in the knee with autologous chondrocyte transplantation. N Engl J Med 331:889–895
5. Brittberg M, Aglietti P, Gambardella R (2001) ICRS cartilage injury evaluation package. International Cartilage Repair Society.
6. Coutts RD, Healey RM, Ostrander R, Sah RL, Goomer R, Amiel D (2001) Matrices for cartilage repair. Clin Orthop 391 [Suppl]:S271–S279
7. Dell'Accio F, De Bari C, Lyuyten FP (2001) Molecular markers predictive of the capacity of expanded human articular chondrocytes to form stable cartilage in vivo. Arthrithis Rheumatism 44:1608–1619
8. Engelhardt M (2002) Das Kniegelenk. Symposium 16.11.2002, Munich, Germany
9. Gaissmaier C, Aicher WK, Fritz J, Weise K (2002) Spender- und kulturabhängige Expression knorpelrelevanter Markergene in humanen artikulären Chondrozyten. Deutsche Gesellschaft für Unfallchirurgie, Jahrestagung, Berlin
10. Kobayashi M, Sakai T, Feige U, Poole RA (2002) A peptide of type II collagen up-regulates gene expression of collagenases and pro-inflammatory cytokines through a MAP-kinas pathway in human chondrocytes. In: Pisetzky DS (ed) ACR, vol 46. Wiley Interscience, New Orleans
11. Micheli LJ, Browne JE, Erggelet C, Fu F, Mandelbaum B, Moseley JB, Zurakowski D (2001) Autologous chondrocyte implantation of the knee: multicenter experience and minimum 3-year follow-up. Clin J Sport Med 11:223–228

12. Mooney DJ, Mikos AG (1999) Growing new organs. Sci Am 280:60–65
13. O'Driscoll SW, Saris DB, Ito Y, Fitzimmons JS (2001) The chondrogenic potential of periosteum decreases with age. J Orthop Res 19:95–103
14. Outerbridge R (1961) The aetiology of chondromalacia patellae. J Bone Joint Surg-Br 43:752
15. Prakash D, Learmonth D (2002) Natural progression of osteo-chondral defect in the femoral condyle. Knee 9:7–10
16. Richardson JB, Caterson B, Evans EH, Ashton BA, Roberts S (1999) Repair of human articular cartilage after implantation of autologous chondrocytes. J Bone Joint Surg-Br 81:1064–1068
17. Sohn DH, Lottman LM, Lum LY, Kim SG, Pedowitz RA, Coutts RD, Sah RL (2002) Effect of gravity on localization of chondrocytes implanted in cartilage defects. Clin Orthop 394:254–262
18. Temenoff JS, Mikos AG (2000) Review: tissue engineering for regeneration of articular cartilage. Biomaterials 21:431–440

Human Mesenchymal Stem Cells: Isolation, Characterization and Chondrogenic Differentiation

15

Ulrich Nöth, Isabella Webering, Susanne Kall, Lars Rackwitz, Jochen Eulert and Rocky S. Tuan

Introduction

Many adult tissues contain populations of stem cells, that have the capacity for tissue regeneration after trauma, disease or aging. The cells may be found within the tissue or in other tissues that serve as stem cell reservoirs. HMSCs (human mesenchymal stem cells) are multipotent progenitor cells, which have the potential to differentiate into a variety of mesenchymal tissues such as bone, cartilage, tendon/ligament, muscle, marrow, fat, and dermis [5, 23]. The cells can be isolated from a variety of tissues using different separation techniques and differentiated into the appropriate phenotype under defined culture conditions, and the action of specific growth factors or cytokines. Characterization of MSCs derived from different tissues has been performed by analyzing their surface marker gene expression profile, but so far no marker exclusively expressed by hMSCs is known.

The chondrogenic differentiation potential of hMSCs is thought to have tremendous clinical implication and might play a key role in future cell-based therapy of articular cartilage defects. Chondrogenesis of MSCs *in vitro* is influenced by a number of factors including a three-dimensional culture format, low oxygen tension and the presence of appropriate growth factors. In high-density pellet cell cultures, in a defined serum-free chondrogenic differentiation medium, and the presence of transforming growth factor β (TGF-β) the chondrogenic differentiation of hMSCs has been established [13, 16, 32]. This pellet cell culture system is a useful system to study the early steps involved in the development of articular cartilage, specifically the formation of extracellular matrix necessary to create a functional cartilage tissue.

Source Tissues, Isolation and Characterization

HMSCs can be isolated from many mesenchymal tissues including bone marrow, periosteum, trabecular bone, adipose tissue, muscle, dermis, blood, and the synovial membrane [5, 7, 11, 14, 18–20, 23, 33, 34]. For all of them it has been shown that they can replicate in an undifferentiated stage *in vitro* and differentiate to cell lineages and tissues of mesenchymal origin. Recent data suggest that the differentiation potential of hMSCs is not restricted to mesenchymal tissues and that the plasticity should be extended to non-mesenchymal tissues of visceral mesodermal, neuroectodermal and endodermal origin [12, 21, 26, 31]. In our department, we have established the isolation of hMSCs derived from bone marrow, adipose tissue, and trabecular bone fragments (Fig. 15.1).

Marrow-Derived Mesenchymal Stem Cells (mhMSCs)

The most common source tissue is bone marrow, which can be easily harvested by a marrow aspiration from the iliac crest with a Yamshidi needle (Fig. 15.1A). Using a density gradient it is possible to separate MSCs from hematopoietic and vascular cells (Fig. 15.1B) [4, 10, 5, 23]. The purified MSCs can be passaged for over 30 population doublings *in vitro* and expanded in number by over one billion-fold without loosing their multipotent differentiation potential [6]. Importantly, there appears to be a decrease in the number of MSCs per total nucleated cells in marrow as a function of age [6]. The addition of fibroblast growth factor-2 (FGF-2) has been shown to increase the growth rate and life span of rabbit, canine, and human bone marrow-derived MSCs in monolayers, without loosing their multipotent mesenchymal differentiation potential [30]. Also, it has been shown that optimal conditions for extensive subcultivation without lineage progression of hMSCs are dependent on the serum lot [15]. Currently, all approaches isolating hMSCs involve whole bone marrow containing a

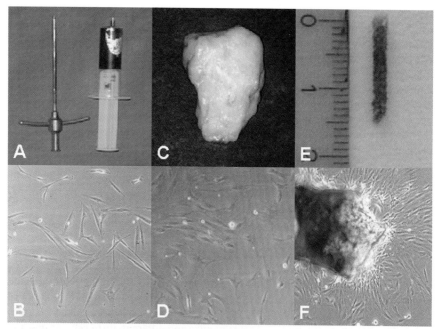

Fig. 15.1A–F. Cell culture of hMSCs derived from different mesenchymal tissues. (**A**) Bone marrow aspirate from the iliac crest using a Yamshidi needle. (**B**) Cell colony of marrow-derived hMSCs at 7 days. (**C**) Fat pad of the knee joint. (**D**) Cell colony of adipose-derived hMSCs at day 10. (**E**) Trabecular bone cylinder harvested from the iliac crest. (**F**) Trabecular bone-derived hMSCs growing out from a collagenase-digested bone fragment at day 14.

low number of MSCs, which can be isolated on their adherence to tissue culture substrates. Most recent data suggest, that the expansion of hMSCs can be significantly increased in suspension bioreactor cultures in the presence of interleukin 3 and steel factor [1].

Adipose Tissue-Derived Mesenchymal Stem Cells (ahMSCs)

Recently, it has been shown that multipotent mesenchymal progenitor cells can be obtained from adipose tissue by suction-assisted lipectomy (i.e. liposuction) [34]. In this technique, the raw lipoaspirate is processed by collagenase digestion to obtain a stromal vascular fraction, which after plating and removal of nonadherent cells is termed processed lipoaspirate [9, 34]. The cells do not appear to require specific serum lots for expansion and differentiation, which has been shown by testing ten different FBS lots from 3 different manufacturers. These cells can be maintained *in vitro* for extended periods with stable population doubling and low levels of senescence. It is known that the stromal vascular fraction processed from the adipose tissue is a heterogeneous cell population including mast cells, endothelial cells, pericytes, fibroblasts, and lineage-committed progenitor cells, or pre-adipocytes [9, 22]. Immunofluorescence and flow cytometry analysis showed that the majority of the cells are of mesenchymal origin with low levels of contaminating pericytes, endothelial cells, and smooth muscle cells [34]. In orthopaedic surgery, primary cultures of adipose tissue-derived hMSCs can be obtained from the fat pad of the knee joint, which can be routinely harvested during total knee arthroplasty (Fig. 15.1C). After mincing, collagenase digestion and plating, the fat pad-derived ahMSCs show a rapidly proliferating homogeneous cell population (Fig. 15.1D).

Trabecular Bone-derived Mesenchymal Stem Cells (bhMSCs)

Cells derived from collagenase-treated human trabecular bone fragments are known to undergo osteoblastic gene expression and matrix mineralization, and are thus considered human osteoblast-like cells [17, 24, 25]. We have recently shown that the cells growing out from the bone fragments have the potential to differentiate into cells of osteogenic, adipogenic and chondrogenic lineages, and functionally resemble mesenchymal stem cells [19]. Most important in this aspect is that collagenase pretreatment of human trabecular bone fragments effectively removes soft tissue components associated with the bone surfaces, such as the periosteum and bone marrow, that may contain heterogeneous cell populations present in variable amounts, depending on the nature of the starting material (gender, donor age and site, amount of red versus yellow marrow, etc.) [25, 25]. Trabecular bone cylinders can be harvested using a Yamshidi needle from the iliac crest (Fig. 15.1E). When the collagenase pretreated bone fragments are cultured as explants in low Ca^{++} growth medium, cells that are surrounded by the mineralized matrix and protected from the collagenasetreatment are subsequently able to migrate from the bone fragments after approximately 2 weeks and begin to proliferate (Fig. 15.1F) [24, 25]. While the origin of the cells is still unclear, they most likely represent osteocytes that have become liberated from their confinement and have once again become mitotic. Some vasculature-associated cells such as pericytes, which have been reported to be able to differentiate into osteoblastic cells, may also contribute to the original cell populations emerging from the bone fragments [3, 17, 25].

Characterization of hMSCs

Cell separation techniques depend on differences in cell density (density gradients using Percoll or Ficoll solutions), affinity of antibodies to cell surface epitopes, (magnetic bead isolation for positive or negative cell sorting) and the fluorescent emission of labeled cells (FACS analysis and flow cytometry). The first 2 techniques involve a relatively low level of technology and are inexpensive, while the third calls for high technology with a significant outlay of capital.

For characterization of hMSCs, flow cytometry analysis using antibodies against specific surface antigens are used (CD = cluster of differentiation). Among others, integrins, hematopoietic markers, cytokine receptors, factor receptors, and matrix receptors are most important. Best characterized are marrow-derived hMSCs from the iliac crest, which have been isolated using a density gradient. These cells represent a cell population, which is uniformly positive (95% to 98%) for the surface antigens SH2, SH3, CD29, CD44, CD71, CD90, CD106, CD120a, and CD124 [23]. The cells also react with the STRO-1 antibody, which binds to an epitope expressed on MSCs. In contrast, the cells are negative for other markers of the hematopoietic lineage, including the lipopolysaccharide receptor CD14, CD34, and the leucocyte common antigen CD45 [23]. Also, a surface protein characterization for human adipose tissue-derived MSCs has been performed. Expressed proteins include CD9, CD10, CD13, CD29, CD34, CD44, CD49, CD54, CD55, CD59, CD105, CD106, CD 146, and CD166 [8]. Unlike human bone marrow-derived MSCs, the STRO-1 antigen is not expressed on human adipose tissue-derived MSCs [8]. Interestingly, these investigators reported that 28% of the cells are CD34-positive. Likewise, human bone marrow-derived MSCs have been described as CD34-positive [29]. These differences might reflect a contamination with cells of the hematopoietic or endothelial lineage. The discrepancies could be also explained by donor heterogeneity, the proliferative stage of the cell culture, the number of passages, the isolation technique used (density gradient or not), different medium composition, and the use of growth factors (e.g. FGF-2). Our own data shows, that trabecular bone-derived hMSCs are positive for CD29, CD44, CD 90, and CD106, and negative for markers of the hematopoietic lineage, including CD34 and the leucocyte common antigen CD45. Table 15.1 summarizes the expression of common surface markers on marrow-derived human MSCs (mhMSCs), adipose tissue-derived human MSCs (ahMSCs), and trabecular bone-derived human MSCs (bhMSCs).

Chondrogenic Differentiation of hMSCs

Understanding the differentiation dependent gene expression of matrix components during chondrogenesis of hMSCs is one of the most important issues for successful hMSC-based articular cartilage repair. The chondrogenic differentiation process *in vit-*

Table 15.1. Surface marker expressed by hMSCs from different source tissues

Antigen	mhMSCs [2] [%]	ahMSCs [30] [%]	bhMSCs (own data) [%]
Positive			
CD 29 (Integrin β1)	>95.0	98.0	96.3
CD 44 (Hyaluronate)	>95.0	60.0	96.7
CD 90 (Thy1)	>95.0	n.t.	95.6
CD 105 (Endoglin)	>95.0	36.0	73.5
Negative			
CD 14 (LPS)	>95.0	99.0	98.4
CD 31 (PECAM-I)	>95.0	99.0	98.4
CD 34 (L-Selectin)	>95.0	72.0	98.9
CD 45 (leukocyt common antigen)	>95.0	99.0	98.1

n.t. = not tested

ro has been established in high-density pellet cell cultures in a serum-free chemically defined differentiation medium containing ascorbate, dexamethasone, sodium pyruvate, proline, ITS-plus, and transforming growth factor (TGF) -β1, -β2 or -β3 [13, 16, 32]. Under these conditions, cell pellets of MSCs developed a cartilage phenotype, characterized by gene expression and synthesis of collagen type II (Coll II), IX (Coll IX), X (Coll X), XI (Coll XI), aggrecan, cartilage proteoglycan link protein, biglycan, decorin, chondroitin 4-sulfate, and keratan sulfate [13, 16, 32]. These chondrogenic cells have been shown to mature further into hypertrophic chondrocytes by the addition of thyroxine, the withdrawal of TGF-β3, and the reduction of dexamethasone [16].

More detailed sequential gene expression analysis leading from the undifferentiated MSC to a mature chondrocyte have been performed for marrow-derived hMSCs [2]. The authors defined 3 separate stages in the differentiation process over a 3-week time period. At an early stage (day 1 to 6) differentiated cells started to express fibromodulin and cartilage oligomeric matrix protein (COMP). An increase in aggrecan, versican core protein, and the small leucine-rich proteoglycans decorin and biglycan defined an intermediate stage (day 6 to 8). This was followed by the appearance of Coll II and chondroadherin at the late stage (day 8 to 21). Coll X, which has an established association with hypertrophic cartilage, was also detected during this differentiation process. Furthermore, less glycaminoclycan and Coll II production was found in cell pellets treated with TGF-β1, when compared to TGF-β2 and -β3 treated pellets, suggesting that both TGF-β2 and TGF-β3 are more effective than TGF-β1.

We have recently shown that trabecular bone-derived hMSCs undergo chondrogenesis when cultured in high-density pellet cultures in the presence of TGF-β1 [19]. As described for marrow-derived hMSCs, pellet cell cultures treated with TGF-β1 increased in size over a 3-week culture period, while omission of TGF-β1 prevented any size increase (Fig. 15.2A,D and G). When stained with haematoxylineosin (HE) TGF-β1 treated pellets showed morphologically distinct, chondrocyte-like cells embedded in extracellular matrix (Fig. 15.2B,C). Staining with alcian blue revealed

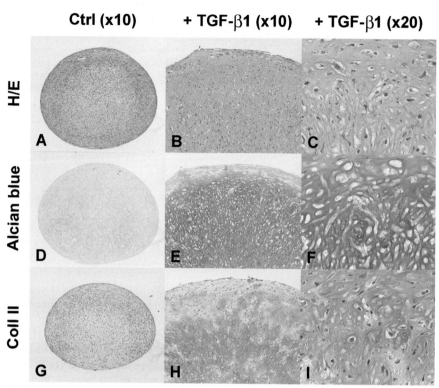

Fig. 15.2A–I. Chondrogenic differentiation of trabecular bone-derived hMSCs cultured in high-density pellet cell cultures for 21 days. (**A–C**) Haematoxylineosin staining. (**D–F**) Alcian blue staining for sulfated proteoglycans. (**G-I**) Immunostaining for collagen type II. Left row shows control cell pellets (Ctrl) treated without TGF-ß1.

that the chondrocyte-like cells were surrounded by a sulfated proteoglycan-rich extracellular matrix (Fig. 15.2E,F) and were rich in Coll II (Fig. 15.2H,I). Furthermore, a sequential gene expression analysis over a 3-week time period using RT-PCR revealed an identical gene expression sequence for Coll II, Coll X, aggrecan, chondroadherin, fibromodulin and COMP, as described for hMSCs (Fig. 15.3).

Conclusion and Future Perspectives

The chondrogenic differentiation potential of MSCs has tremendous clinical implication. The TGF-β induced chondrogenesis of hMSCs *in vitro* involves the rapid expression of cartilage-specific genes and the deposition of cartilage-specific extracellular matrix. There are parallels between this *in vitro* differentiation and the chondrogenic process following mesenchymal condensation during development of the fetal limb, such as the expression of chondroadherin and collagen type II, which is low in immature cartilage and increases with maturation [27, 28]. The appearance and functional

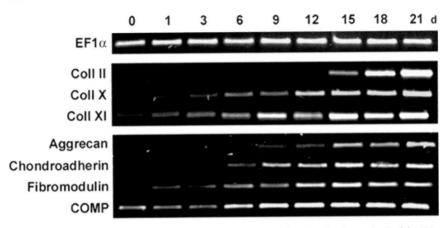

Fig. 15.3. RT-PCR analysis of chondrogenic marker genes of trabecular bone-derived hMSCs during chondrogenic differentiation in the presence of TGF-ß1 for 21 days.

role of collagen type X which is thought to be unique to mature hypertrophic cartilage in the growth plate and is only found elsewhere under pathological conditions, e. g. osteoarthritic articular cartilage and chondrosarcoma, is unknown. In conclusion, more detailed *in vitro* investigations are needed to understand the pathways and define the events during chondrogenesis leading from the undifferentiated MSC to the mature chondrocyte. These data are essential to develop successful mesenchymal stem cell-based strategies for future articular cartilage repair.

References

1. Baksh D, Zandstra BW, Davies JE (2002) Expansion of human osteogenic progenitors in stirred suspension bioreactors. Trans Orthop Res Soc 48:542
2. Barry F, Boynton RE, Liu B, Murphy JM (2001) Chondrogenic differentiation of mesenchymal stem cells from bone marrow: differentiation-dependent gene expression of matrix components. Exp Cell Res 268:189–200
3. Brighton CT, Lorich DG, Kupcha R, Reilly TM, Jones AR, Woodbury RA (1990) The pericyte as a possible osteoblast progenitor cell. Clin Orthop 275:287–299
4. Bruder SP, Kurth AA, Shea M, Hayes WC, Jaiswal N, Kadiyala S (1998) Bone regeneration by implantation of purified, culture-expanded human mesenchymal stem cells. J Orthop Res 16:155–162
5. Caplan AI (1994) The mesengenic process. Clin Plast Surg 21:429–435
6. Caplan AI, Bruder SP (1997) Cell and molecular engineering of bone regeneration. In: Lanza RP, Langer R, Chick WL (eds) Principles of tissue engineering. Academic Press, San Diego, pp603–618
7. De Bari C, Dell'Accio F, Tylzanowski P, Luyten FP (2001) Multipotent mesenchymal stem cells from adult human synovial membrane. Arthritis Rheum 44:1928–1942
8. Gronthos S, Franklin DM, Leddy HA, Robey PG, Storms RW, Gimble JM (2001) Surface protein characterization of human adipose tissue-derived stromal cells. J Cell Physiol 189:54–63
9. Hauner H, Schmid P, Pfeiffer EF (1987) Glucocorticoids and insulin promote the differentiation of human adipocyte precorsor cells into fat cells. J Clin Endocrinol Meatbol 64:832–835

10. Haynesworth SE, Goshima J, Goldberg VM, Caplan AI (1992) Characterization of cells with osteogenic potential from human marrow. Bone 13:81–88
11. Jankowski RJ, Deasy BM, Huard J (2002) Muscle-derived stem cells. Gene Therapy 9:642–647
12. Jiang Y, Jahagirdar BN, Reinhardt RL et al. (2002) Pluripotency of mesenchymal stem cells derived from adult marrow. Nature 418:41–49
13. Johnstone B, Hering MH, Caplan AI, Goldberg VM, Yoo JU (1998) In vitro chondrogenesis of bone marrow-derived mesenchymal progenitor cells. Exp Cell Res 238:265–272
14. Kutznetsov SA, Mankani MH, Gronthos S, Satomura K, Bianco P, Robey P (2001) Circulating skeletal stem cells. J Cell Biology 5:1133–1140
15. Lennon DP, Haynesworth SE, Young RG, Dennis JE, Caplan A (1995) Chemically defined medium supports in vitro proliferation and maintains the osteochondral potential of rat marrow-derived mesenchymal stem cells. Exp Cell Res 219:211–222
16. Mackay AM, Beck SC, Murphy JM, Barry FP, Chichester CO, Pittenger MF (1998) Chondrogenic differentiation of cultured human mesenchymal stem cells from marrow. Tissue Eng 4:415–428
17. Majeska RJ (1996) Culture of osteoblastic cells. In: Bilezikian JP, Raisz LG, Rodan GA (eds) Principles of bone biology. Academic Press, San Diego, pp1229–1238
18. Nakahara H, Bruder SP, Haynesworth SE, Holecek JJ, Baber MA, Goldberg VM, Caplan AI (1990) Bone and cartilage formation in diffusion chambers by subcultured cells derived from periosteum. Bone 11:181–188
19. Nöth U, Osyczka AM, Tuli R, Hickok NJ, Danielson KG, Tuan RS (2002) Multilineage differentiation potential of human trabecular bone-derived cells. J Orthop Res 20:1060–1069
20. Nöth U, Tuli R, Osyczka AM, Danielson KG, Tuan RS (2002) In vitro engineered cartilage constructs produced by press-coating biodegradable polymer with human mesenchymal stem cells. Tissue Eng 8:131–143
21. Oh SH, Miyazaki M, Kouchi H et al. (2000) Hepatocyte growth factor induces differentiation of adult rat bone marrow cells into a hepatocyte lineage in vitro. Biochem Biophys Res Commun 279:500–504
22. Pettersson P, Cigolini M, Sjoestroem L, Smith U, Bjoerntrop P (1985) Cells in human adipose tissue developing into adipocytes. Acta Med Scand 215:447–451
23. Pittenger MF, Mackay AM, Beck SC (1999) Multilineage potential of adult human mesenchymal stem cells. Science 284:143–147
24. Robey PG (1995) Collagenase-treated trabecular bone fragments: a reproducible source of cells in the osteoblastic lineage. Calcif Tissue Int 56 [Suppl 1]:S11–S12
25. Robey PG, Termine JD (1985) Human bone cells in vitro. Calcif Tissue Int 37:453–460
26. Sanchez-Ramos J, Song S, Cardozo-Pelaez F et al. (2000) Adult bone marrow stromal cells differentiate into neural cells in vitro. Exp Neurol 164:247–256
27. Sandberg M, Vuorio E (1987) Localization of types I, II, and III collagen mRNAs in developing human skeletal tissues by in situ hybridization. J Cell Biol 104:1077–1084
28. Shen Z, Gantcheva S, Mansson B, Heinegard D, Sommarin Y (1998) Chondroadherin expression changes in skeletal development. Biochem J 330:549–457
29. Simmons PJ, Torok-Storb B (1991) CD34 expression by stromal precursors in normal human adult bone marrow. Blood 78:2848–2853
30. Tsutsumi S, Shimazu A, Miyazaki K et al. (2001) Retention of multilineage differentiation potential of mesenchymal cells during proliferation in response to FGF. Biochem Biophys Res Commun 288:413–419
31. Woodbury D, Schwarz EJ, Prockop DJ, Black IB (2000) Adult rat and human bone marrow stromal cells differentiate into neurons. J Neurosci Res 61:364–370
32. Yoo JU, Barthel TS, Nishimura K, Solchaga L, Caplan AI, Goldberg VM, Johnstone B (1998) The chondrogenic potential of human bone marrow-derived mesenchymal progenitor cells. J Bone Joint Surg-A 80:1745–1757
33. Young HE, Steele TA, Bray RA et al. (2001) Human reserve pluripotent mesenchymal stem cells are present in the connective tissues of skeletal muscle and dermis derives from fetal, adult, and geriatric donors. Anatomical Record 264:51–62
34. Zuk PA, Zhu M, Mizuno H et al. (2001) Multilineage cells from human adipose tissue: implication for cell-based therapies. Tissue Eng 7:211–228

Experimental in Vivo Results

Chondrocytes and Polymer Fleeces* 16

MAXIMILIAN RUDERT

Introduction

Different surgical techniques have been introduced as treatment options for chondral and osteochondral defects [31]. Apart from debridement or chondroplasty, opening of the marrow cavity is used to induce bleeding and to initiate the formation of fibrocartilaginous scar tissue. More recent techniques have tried to implement some type of biological surface repair. These treatments include the transplantation of chondrogenic materials such as periosteum [14], or perichondrium [3], as well as chondrocyte transplantation as a suspension [2], or the transplantation of tissue-engineered cartilage constructs [1, 6, 8–10, 13, 16, 18, 27, 29, 30]. Promising results have been reported and many investigators have focused their efforts on the creation of a more natural hyaline cartilage using isolated chondrocytes or mesenchymal stem cells on different types of carrier materials. Only a small piece of original cartilage must be sacrificed in order to propagate the number of cells *in vitro,* and to create a new cartilaginous matrix for implantation into a large defect. Maturation of the tissue *in vitro* is appealing because cartilage-specific matrix can be remodeled by the immobilized cultured cells before transplantation (Fig. 16.1). Various materials have been used in different experimental animals but a comparison of different carrier matrices cultured with chondrocytes in the same experimental set-up has not been carried out so far. We therefore investigated 3 resorbable matrices in an osteochondral defect model in the rabbit knee. The investigated matrices have previously been found suitable for the creation of tissue-engineered cartilage *in vitro* [21–23].

Material and Methods

Thirty-three 5 to 6 months old female New Zealand white rabbits weighting between 3.5 and 5.5 kg were used. The rabbits were randomly treated with one of the carrier matrices with or without cultured chondrocytes, or were simply left empty to serve as controls. Up to 3 defect locations were scheduled for each knee: the trochlear groove, and the medial and lateral condyle. Care was taken not to apply 2 different materials

* This study was funded in part by grants from the Deutsche Forschungsgemeinschaft (DFG, Wi 494/14–1) and by the Deutsche Arthrose Hilfe.

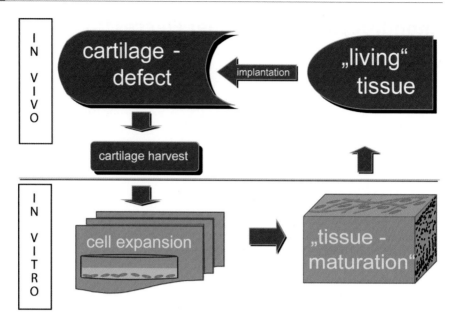

Fig. 16.1. Schematic drawing of the tissue engineering process from defect to repair.

in one knee. Prior to transplantation, allogenic chondrocytes were harvested from the knees of 3 to 5 months old female New Zealand white rabbits, which were sacrificed for another unrelated study. Chondrocytes were isolated enzymatically, expanded in monolayer culture and seeded on 3 different three-dimensional carrier materials as previously described [21]. Animal experiments were approved by the ethics commitee of the District Government of Lower Saxony.

Two synthetic resorbable polymer fleeces, Ethisorb® 210 and PLLA (poly-L-lactic acid), were compared with lyophilized dura as a biological fleece material. These fleece materials are well known in the field of surgery and have been approved for human use.

- Ethisorb® 210 (Ethicon, Norderstedt, Germany) is a polydioxanon/polygalactin polymer.
- PLLA (V19–1; Institute for Textile Technology and Process Engineering, Denk-endorf, Germany) is a poly-L-lactic acid fleece.
- Lyophilized dura (B. Braun-Dexon; Spangenberg, Germany) is mainly composed of collagen type I. Soaked in suspension the 2 leafs of the dura can easily be separat-ed leaving 2 fleece layers with a smooth and dense layer on one surface.

The materials were cut into individual discs measuring 3×3 mm prior to incubation with isolated chondrocytes. After 4 weeks of three-dimensional culture, the cell-carri-er constructs were implanted. All operations were performed under sterile conditions with the animals under general anesthesia. Three mm full-thickness defects were cre-ated with a handdrill in the most posterior part of the medial and lateral condyles as well as in the center of the trochlear groove. The defects were drilled until small bleeding points were visible at the bottom of the defects. The defect was either left empty, filled with one of the carrier materials only, or filled with a carrier material cultured with cells. These materials were press-fitted into the defects.

In 33 animals a total of 101 defects was created. Thirty-eight defects were followed over 6 weeks, 27 defects over 6 months, and 36 defects for up to 12 months. The synovium of the retrieved samples was observed for signs of inflammation. The joint itself was inspected for osteophyte formation indicating degeneration.

Macroscopic evaluation was done with a score, and a maximum of 8 points and a minimum of 3 points were assigned according to the degree of the defect-filling:
- distinct underneath surrounding cartilage,
- up to surrounding cartilage, central depression,
- flush with surrounding cartilage;

the defect color:
- brown or yellow,
- white,
- cartilaginous, same as surrounding cartilage;

and the surface integrity of the repair tissue:
- rough,
- smooth.

For the microscopic evaluation, defects including the surrounding cartilage and bone were fixed in 4% para-formaldehyde, decalcified with EDTA, and embedded in paraffin (n = 101). Sections (5 μm) were cut and stained with safranin O and toluidine blue, while randomly selected specimens were stained with alcian blue, at a pH = 1.0, in order to detect sulfated glycosaminoglycans. Histological sections from the central portion of each defect were evaluated independently by 3 investigators according to the O'Driscoll score [15] and a maximum of 24 points could be achieved.

Histochemical evaluation of collagen types I and II were carried out with monoclonal antibodies against collagen type I (COL 1, mouse IgG1, C2456, Sigma; 1:500) [26] and collagen type II (CIIC1, mouse IgG2a, Developmental Studies Hybridoma Bank, Iowa, USA; 1:20) [19] using the DAB-method. Sections were dewaxed in xylol, treated with 0.1% pepsin in 0.5 mol acetic acid and hyaluronidase at 37 °C. To reduce endogenous peroxidase activity, 0.6% H_2O_2-methanol was applied. Slides were incubated with the first antibody for 60 min in a moist chamber, followed by PAP anti-mouse (Dako, 1:200, 30 min). Peroxidase was visualized with the DAB substratekit (3,3'-diaminobenzidine, Serva, Heidelberg). Controls were first imaged without the first antibody. The results were scored as follows: no collagen staining = 0; collagen type stained area less than 50% of the defect area = 1; collagen type stained area more than 50% of defect area = 2; collagen type stained area approximately 100% = 3 points.

Statistical analysis was performed using the Tukey-HSD *post hoc* test for individual differences (statistical significance was set at α = 0.05). All tests were performed using of SPSS for Windows.

Results

No complications were seen during the operation or in the postoperative period. There was no evidence of joint inflammation or gross abnormalities in any of the articulating surfaces. No significant differences were detected between any of the experimental groups, regardless of the follow-up time, applying the macroscopic scoring system. After 6 weeks most of the defects were filled to the level of the surrounding cartilage, but had a more whitish appearance than the surrounding cartilage (Fig. 16.2). Especially in the 12-month group, the results of the control defect looked very good. This finding did not correspond to the results of the microscopic score.

The results of the microscopic evaluation showed large variability, ranging from a minimum score of 3 points to a maximum score of 21, out of the possible 24 points.

All matrices reached comparable results with scores between 11.5 and 12.7 points (equivalent to 48% to 53% of the possible 24 points) at 6 weeks. Only the defects treated with dura and cells reached a score of 16.4 points (68%). The untreated control defects had the lowest score of only 10.3 points (43%). After 6 months, the differences between the defects seeded with cells and the group treated with carriers

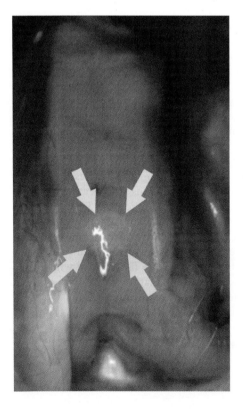

Fig. 16.2.
Photomicrograph of a 3 mm trochlear defect treated with dura cultured with cells 6 weeks after implantation in the rabbit knee. The defect area is still visible (*arrows*). Defect filling can be described as flush with surrounding cartilage. The defect color is white and the surface integrity of the repair tissue is smooth (7/8 points of the macroscopic score).

alone increased. Again, the best results were achieved by the defects treated with dura plus cells (16.6 points, 69%), followed by the defects treated with PLLA and cells (64%), and Ethisorb® with cells (62%). If only the carriers were implanted, the results were considerably inferior (35% for PLLA, 45% for Ethisorb®, and 51% for dura). The cell-free control specimens reached an average score of 12.8 points (54%) at 6 months. This was also seen in the 12-month specimens. Regardless of the applied carrier material, defects treated with cultured cells provided superior results (dura: 15.3 points, 64%; Ethisorb®: 15.2 points, 63%; PLLA: 15 points, 63%) compared to the cell-free defects treated only with the carrier (PLLA: 7.0 points, 29%, dura: 9.2 points, 38%; Ethisorb®: 12.3 points, 51%) or the empty control defects (11.8 points, 49%).

A significant effect could be obtained through the addition of cultured cells (p <0.0005) as compared to the cell-free carrier materials alone. There was also a significant difference between the cell group and the empty controls (p <0.002), but not between the carrier group and the empty controls (p <0.842).

The amount of collagen types I and II could be quantified estimating the percentage of the stained defect area, revealing an increase of type II in the cell group over time (p <0.005), and a decrease in the collagen type I content (p <0.0005), compared to the cell-free carrier controls (p <0.005 for collagen type II, p <0.0005). A seamless repair could not be achieved (Fig. 16.3 and Fig. 16.4).

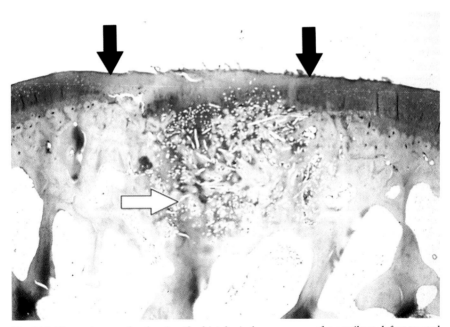

Fig. 16.3. Photomicrographs showing the histological appearance of a cartilage defect treated with a cell-seeded PLLA fleece after 12 month (safranin-O, ×2.5). Remnants of the PLLA fibers can be distinguished in the defect area (*white arrow*). At the borders of the defect a good integration of the transplanted tissue is visible on one side, whereas a small cleft formation is evident on the other side.

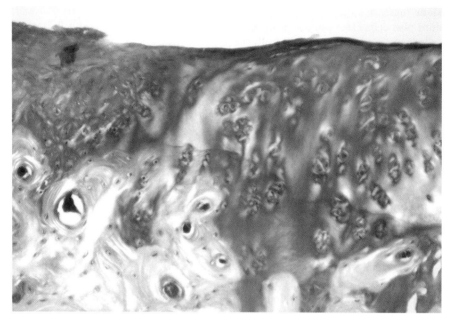

Fig. 16.4. Under polarized light a good integration of the collagen fibers of the implanted material (*left*) to the host cartilage (*right*) can be observed (safranin-O polarized light, ×12.5).

Discussion

One of the pre-requisites for the creation of bioartificial or tissue engineered cartilage *in vitro* is the use of a carrier matrix which can serve as a three-dimensional scaffold to anchor the amplified cells [7]. On the scaffold the cells start the production of cartilage-specific matrix *in vitro* [23] before they are implanted into a cartilage defect. We compared 3 biodegradable carrier materials for isolated chondrocytes, which already had the opportunity to re-differentiate *in vitro* [4, 5, 28] and produce a significant amount of cartilage specific matrix [23].

Shapiro et al. described impressive early positive results for 3 mm osteochondral defects in a similar repair model. However, degenerative changes were observed to an increasing extent after 48 weeks in these animals [25]. Shagaldi et al. investigated the repair of cartilage defects with different biological materials in goats. They reported an increased onset of degeneration of the repairs 12 months after the initial operation [24]. Therefore, a maximum follow-up period of 56 weeks was chosen in the presented study to allow the evaluation of early degenerative changes [20].

The results of the macroscopic evaluation in our study were not constant and did not correlate to the microscopic result. Good macroscopic appearance could be associated with an inferior microscopic score. This observation seems noteworthy, because of the fact that macroscopic evaluation of defect repair is commonly employed during arthroscopic procedures.

Interestingly, the microscopic evaluation of the repaired defect revealed no statistical differences between the different carrier matrices used. One would expect differences in the material properties of the to have a detectable influence on the resulting defect repair. The tendency of the carrier dura to provide slightly superior microscopic results might be due to the bi-layer composition of this material. The superficial network of collagen fibers resembles a fleece-like material, that is suitable for anchoring the isolated cells. The deep and dense layer of the material creates a barrier to the underlying marrow space of the osteochondral defect. This could have an inhibitory effect on the invasion of pluripotent cells from the marrow cavity into the defect, which on its own can lead to the creation of fibrocartilage. We could recently demonstrate the survival of implanted cells, by retroviral infection with green fluorescent protein, for at least four weeks *in vivo*. Therefore, a complete replacement of implanted cells by mesenchymal stem cells from the marrow cavity is unlikely [11,30].

The addition of isolated chondrocytes to carrier matrices *in vitro,* and the transplantation of these cultured constructs into the defect significantly improved healing of osteochondral defects. These results did not statistically depend on the duration of the experiment. To evaluate the histological results we prefer the scoring system introduced by O'Driscoll [15]. This score includes degenerative changes and is therefore suitable for long-term evaluation of osteochondral defect repair, in contrast to other histological scores that are easier to use [17, 20, 29]. While collagen type II content increased over time, collagen type I content was decreased. Unfortunately, in most of the defects collagen type I could still be detected, even after 56 weeks. The detection of collagen type I implies that we are still dealing with some sort of fibrocartilaginous tissue. Breinan et al. investigated the effect of chondrocyte seeded on collagen type II matrices in a chondral defect model in 15 dogs. The results were compared to microfractured (osteochondral) defects and to microfractured defects treated with a collagen type II matrix without the addition of cells. After 15 weeks they found predominantly fibrocartilage, without any significant differences between their treatment groups [1].

Comparison of the different bioresorbable carrier materials in our study did not reveal a significant influence of the bioartificial cartilage construct material on the result of osteochondral defect repair. Interestingly, the addition of cells to the carrier materials led to a significant improvement of the histological score, as well as the ratio of collagen type I and II. Although this improvement is significant, the overall result of 16 out of 24 possible points of the histological scoring system is still not satisfying. In a recent publication by Im et al. a mean score of 14.8 points was attained through the application of autologous mesenchymal stem cells from bone marrow aspirates in a 3 mm osteochondral defects, which were then covered with a fascia lata flap in a rabbit model. They observed a large variability in the results of the experimental group, as well as the control group, and attributed this to technical failures and to individual differences in the capability of self-repair [12].

We observed a significant improvement of the histological scoring system evaluating osteochondral defect repair when cells were added to the implanted materials, although no difference could be observed between the different materials. The results are promising, but before this technique is applied in human we still need to improve the quality of the repair.

References

1. Breinan HA, Martin SD, Hsu HP, Spector M (2000) Healing of canine articular cartilage defects treated with microfracture, a type-II collagen matrix, or cultured autologous chondrocytes. J Orthop Res 18:781–789
2. Brittberg M, Lindahl A, Nilsson A, Ohlsson C, Isaksson O, Peterson L (1994) Treatment of deep cartilage defects in the knee with autologous chondrocyte transplantation. N Engl J Med 331:889–895
3. Bruns J, Kersten P, Lierse W, Silbermann M (1992) Autologous rib perichondral grafts in experimentally induced osteochondral lesions in the sheep knee joint: morphological results. Virchows Arch 421:1–8
4. Daniels K, Solursh M (1991) Modulation of chondrogenesis by the cytoskeleton and extracellular matrix. J Cell Science 100:249–254
5. Domm C, Fay J, Schünke M, Kurz B (2000) Die Redifferenzierung von dedifferenzierten Gelenkknorpelzellen in Alginatkultur. Einfluss von intermittierendem hydrostatischen Druck und niedrigem Sauerstoffpartialdruck. Orthopäde 29:91–99
6. Freed LE, Grande DA, Lingbin Z, Emmanual J, Marquis JC, Langer R (1994) Joint resurfacing using allograft chondrocytes and synthetic biodegradable polymer scaffolds. J Biomed Mater Res 28:891–899
7. Freed LE, Marquis JC, Nohria JC, Emmanual J, Mikos AG, Langer R (1993) Neocartilage formation in vitro and in vivo using cells cultured on synthetic biodegradable polymers. J Biomed Mater Res 27:11–23
8. Frenkel SR, Toolan BC, Menche D, Pitman MI, Pachence JM (1997) Chondrocyte transplantation using a collagen bilayer matrix for cartilage repair. J Bone Joint Surg-Br 79:831–836
9. Helbing G (1982) Transplantation isolierter Chondrozyten in Gelenkknorpel-Defekte. Fortschr Med 100:83–87
10. Hendrickson DA, Nixon AJ, Grande DA, Todhunter RJ, Minor RM, Erb H, Lust G (1994) Chondrocyte-fibrin matrix transplants for resurfacing extensive articular cartilage defects. J Orthop Res 12:485–497
11. Hirschmann F, Verhoeyen E, Wirth D, Bauwens S, Hauser H, Rudert M (2002) Vital marking of articular chondrocytes by retroviral infection using green fluorescence protein. Osteoarthritis Cartilage 10:109–118
12. Im GI, Kim DY, Shin JH, Hyun CW, Cho WH (2001) Repair of cartilage defect in the rabbit with cultured mesenchymal stem cells from bone marrow. J Bone Joint Surg-Br 83:289–294
13. Nehrer S, Breinan HA, Ramappa A et al. (1998) Chondrocyte-seeded collagen matrices implanted in a chondral defect in a canine model. Biomaterials 19:2313–2328
14. O'Driscoll SW (1999) Articular cartilage regeneration using periosteum. Clin Orthop 367 [Suppl]:S186–S203
15. O'Driscoll SW, Keeley FW, Salter RB (1988) Durability of regenerated articular cartilage produced by free autogenous periosteal grafts in major full-thickness defects in joint surfaces under the influence of continuous passive motion. A follow-up report at one year. J Bone Joint Surg-A 70:595–606
16. Perka C, Schultz O, Sittinger M, Zippel H (2000) Chondrozytentransplantation in PGLA Polydioxanon-Vliesen. Orthopäde 29:112–119
17. Pineda S, Pollack A, Stevenson S, Goldberg VM, Caplan AI (1992) A semiquantitative scale for histologic grading of articular cartilage repair. Acta Anat 143:335–340
18. Rahfoth B, Weisser J, Sternkopf F, Aigner T, von der M, Brauer R (1998) Transplantation of allograft chondrocytes embedded in agarose gel into cartilage defects of rabbits. Osteoarthritis Cartilage 6:50–65
19. Ramdi H, Tahri-Jouti MA, Lievremont M (1993) Immobilized articular chondrocytes: in vitro production of extracellular matrix compounds. Biomat Artif Cells Immob Biotech 21:335–341
20. Rudert M (2002) Histological evaluation of osteochondral defects: consideration of animal models with emphasis on the rabbit, experimental setup, follow-up and applied methods. Cells Tissues Organs 171:229–240

21. Rudert M, Hirschmann F, Schulze M, Wirth CJ (2000) Bioartificial cartilage. Cells Tissues Organs 167:95–105
22. Rudert M, Hirschmann F, Wirth CJ (1999) Wachstumsverhalten von Chondrozyten auf unterschiedlichen Trägersubstanzen. Orthopäde 28:68–75
23. Rudert M, Wirth CJ, Schulze M, Reiss G (1998) Synthesis of articular cartilage like tissue in vitro. Arch Orthop Trauma Surg 117:141–146
24. Shahgaldi BF, Amis AA, Heatley FW, McDowell J, Bentley G (1991) Repair of cartilage lesions using biological implants. A comparative histological and biomechanical study in goats. J Bone Joint Surg-Br 73:57–64
25. Shapiro F, Koide S, Glimcher MJ (1993) Cell origin and differentiation in the repair of full-thickness defects of articular cartilage. J Bone Joint Surg-A 75:532–553
26. Sittinger M, Bujia J, Minuth WW, Hammer C, Burmester GR (1994) Engineering of cartilage tissue using bioresorbable polymer carriers in perfusion culture. Biomaterials 15:451–456
27. Vacanti CA, Kim WS, Schloo B, Upton J, Vacanti JP (1994) Joint resurfacing with cartilage grown in situ from cell-polymer structures. Am J Sports Med 22:485–488
28. von der Mark K (1986) Differentiation, modulation and dedifferentiation of chondrocytes. Rheumatology 10:272–315
29. Wakitani S, Goto T, Pineda SJ, Young RG, Mansour JM, Caplan AI, Goldberg VM (1994) Mesenchymal cell-based repair of large, full-thickness defects of articular cartilage. J Bone Joint Surg-A 76:579–592
30. Weisser J, Rahfoth B, Timmermann A, Aigner T, Bräuer R, von der Mark K (2001) Role of growth factors in rabbit articular cartilage repair by chondrocytes in agarose. Osteoarthritis Cartilage 9 [Suppl A]:48–54
31. Wirth CJ, Rudert M (1996) Techniques of cartilage growth enhancement: a review of the literature. Arthroscopy 12:300–308

CHAPTER 17

Chondrocytes and Fibrin Glue*   17

CARSTEN PERKA, SEBASTIAN STERN, RON-SASCHA SPITZER
and KLAUS LINDENHAYN

Introduction

Growth, morphology and differentiation of cells *in vitro* depend on the composition of the cellular environment. Therefore, a variety of matrices have been studied to provide optimal conditions for chondrocyte culture. The introduction of alginate as a supporting matrix into cell culture was a blessing for cells that need to be cultured in a three-dimensional matrix. Alginate, a linear polysaccharide, is a co-polymer of two uronic acids: L-guluronic and D-mannuronic acid linked by 1 to 4 glycosidic bonds. The polymer undergoes instantaneous ionotrophic gelation in the presence of divalent cations, e.g. calcium. Compared to other gel matrices, alginate beads offer a simple way of dissolution to the monomer subunits using chelating agents, such as sodium citrate, releasing the entrapped cells together with their synthesized high molecular matrix.

Due to the ongoing discussion on the composition of the alginates concerning their biocompatibility, new strategies for three-dimensional cell cultivation have to be examined. This chapter describes the technique for the preparation of pure and mixed fibrin beads for tissue engineering. In mixed alginate-fibrin beads, the alginate ratio of the beads has to be extracted before implantation due to its lack of biodegradability. The presence of alginate is only necessary for the exact formation of the composite beads.

Materials and Methods

Preparation of Fibrin-alginate Beads, Fibrin Beads, and Fibrin-hyaluronic acid Beads

Two hundred µL of 4.8% alginate (Sigma, St Louis, MO, USA) in isotonic sodium chloride (see [2]), 500 µL fibrinogen (Fibrin glue Beriplast® HS, Centeon Pharma GmbH, Marburg, Germany), and 100 µL cell suspension, in 140 mM NaCl, 5 mM KCl, 10 mM HEPES, 10 mM glucose, 0.02% EDTA were mixed thoroughly in a small siliconized glass vial. The cell suspension was dropped (Eppendorf pipette, yellow tip) slowly into a mixture of 10 mL 102 mM calcium chloride and 1 mL thrombin (Beriplast® HS).

---

* This work was supported by a grant of the Steinbeis-Foundation and the DFG (Deutsche Forschungsgemeinschaft).

During pipetting, the vial containing the cell suspension has to be kept in motion to achieve an homogeneous distribution of the cells in the beads. Subsequently, the beads were allowed to polymerize in the calcium chloride/thrombin solution for 20 min at room temperature. The beads were washed twice with 140 mM NaCl, 5 mM KCl, 10 mM HEPES, 10 mM glucose, and 0.02% EDTA.

For preparation of pure fibrin beads, the alginate was extracted from the alginate fibrin beads by a solution of 55 mM sodium citrate, 150 mM NaCl, and 30 mM EDTA (pH 6.8) for 15 min [2]. Then, the beads were washed sequentially once with 0.16 M NaCl and twice with DMEM/Ham's F-12 (1:1)/HEPES pH = 7.3.

For cultivation of nucleus pulposus cells a mixture of fibrinogen and hyaluronic acid for gel preparation was used. Therefore, the cell pellet was suspended in isotonic sodium chloride containing fibrinogen mixed with hyaluronic acid (Hy-GAG®, Chemedica, Munich, Germany) to reach a final concentration of fibrinogen by 2.25% and hyaluronic acid by 0.33%.

Fibrin-alginate beads, fibrin-hyaluronic acid beads, and fibrin beads containing cells were cultured in roller bottles (diameter 110 mm, length 171 mm, Reichelt Chemietechnik GmbH, Heidelberg, Germany) in DMEM/Ham's F-12 containing 10% FCS. Dissolution of the fibrin beads during culturing could be inhibited by supplementation of the culture medium with 240 to 500 KIE/mL of aprotinin (Trasylol®, Bayer Vital GmbH, Leverkusen, Germany).

Results and Discussion

Common tissue engineering principles focus on following essential components: functionally active cells, which have to be non-immunogenic, easy to achieve, and highly responsive to differential environmental cues, an appropriate carrier for *in vitro* differentiation and subsequent transplantation, and a set of defined bioactive molecules initiating the process of differentiation and maturation.

Using this fibrin bead culture model, we have cultured chondrocytes [1, 5], periosteal-derived cells [3, 4, 6], and nucleus pulposus cells [7, 8]. We cultivated chondrocytes in alginate and in fibrin-alginate beads, and found a significantly higher cell proliferation in the composite fibrin-alginate beads [3]. For the preparation of fibrin-containing alginate beads we dropped an alginate-fibrinogen mixture containing cells into a solution of calcium chloride and thrombin. Calcium ions "polymerize" the alginate chains, whereas thrombin transforms the soluble fibrinogen into insoluble fibrin. If needed, the alginate can be removed at any time from the fibrin-alginate beads by sodium citrate leaving spherical fibrin beads containing cells. Chondrocytes maintained their typical spherical morphology throughout the culture period in fibrin-alginate gels in contrast to cells cultured in pure fibrin beads where chondrocytes dedifferentiated into fibroblast-like cells [3]. Furthermore, the synthesis of specific matrix components was evident in mixed fibrin-alginate beads (Fig. 17.1).

Periosteal-derived cells in fibrin beads containing 7.5% α-tricalcium phosphate (α-TCP, 120 to 230 mesh) have shown a higher cell proliferation in comparison to fibrin beads without α-TCP [6]. Histological analysis of the beads indicated that distribution of periosteal-derived cells changed during the culture period from a homogeneous to a more surface-orientated distribution (Fig. 17.2). Furthermore, fibrin beads can be used to investigate the influence of different growth factors like TGF-β, b-FGF, or factor XIII on proliferation and differentiation of periosteal-derived cells [6].

Composite fibrin-hyaluronic acid beads are also suitable for the culture of cells from nucleus pulposus, where we found a higher ³⁵S-sulfate incorporation related to cell number in comparison to alginate alone (Fig. 17.3) [7]. The combination of fibrin

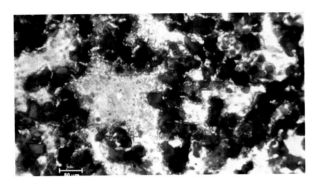

Fig. 17.1.
Immunolocalization of cartilage proteoglycan in sections of fibrin-alginate beads containing human chondrocytes (×400).

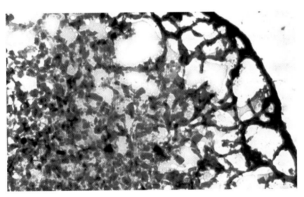

Fig. 17.2.
Homogeneous distribution of human periosteal-derived cells in fibrin beads (MG, ×200).

Fig. 17.3.
Immunolocalization of pericellular accumulated proteoglycan in sections of fibrin-hyaluronic acid beads containing porcine nucleus pulposus cells (×200).

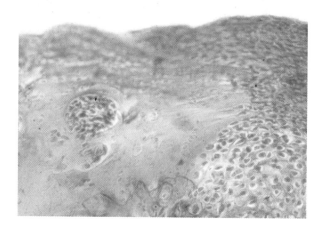

Fig. 17.4.
Hyaline cartilage 3 weeks after implantation of rabbit chondrocytes. The defect is completely filled by the implant (HE, ×100).

with hyaluronic acid prevents the substantial loss of hyaluronic acid from the culture system [1]. The hyaluronic acid was added as cells can adhere to the macromolecule via the CD44-receptor, thereby directly affecting the cellular function and cytoskeletal structure. Using this composite matrix, even the cultivation of nucleus pulposus cells from degenerated intervertebral disc cells was possible [8].

An advantage is the simple and secure *in vivo* fixation of fibrin beads in cartilage, osteochondral and bone defects (Fig. 17.4) [4,5]. For instance, we used periosteal-derived cells cultured in fibrin beads for successful reconstruction of critical-sized bone defects in NZW rabbits [5].

In conclusion, we think that the fibrin beads are effective carrier structures in supporting the bone- and cartilage-forming potential of different types of cells. Alginate can serve as a temporary supportive matrix component during *in vitro* culture and can easily be removed prior to transplantation to circumvent the problem of missing biodegradability of alginates and to improve cell nutrition. Therefore, it seems to be useful to combine different matrices and their advantages for cell culture. Our method could be of great value for the culture of other cell types as well.

References

1. Lindenhayn K, Perka C, Spitzer RS, Heilmann HH, Pommerening K, Mennicke J, Sittinger M (1999) Retention of hyaluronic acid in alginate beads: aspects for in vitro cartilage engineering. J Biomed Mater Res 44:149–155
2. Mok SS, Masuda K, Häuselmann HJ, Aydelotte MB, Thonar EJMA (1994) Aggrecan synthesized by mature bovine chondrocytes suspended in alginate. J Biol Chem 269:33021–33027
3. Perka C, Schultz O, Spitzer RS, Lindenhayn K (2000) The influence of transforming growth factor β1 on mesenchymal cell repair of full-thickness cartilage defects. J Biomed Mater Res 52:543–552

4. Perka C, Schultz O, Spitzer RS, Lindenhayn K, Burmester GR, Sittinger M (2000) Segmental bone repair by tissue engineered periosteal cell transplants with bioresorbable fleece and fibrin scaffolds in rabbits. Biomaterials 21:1145–1153

5. Perka C, Spitzer RS, Lindenhayn K, Sittinger M, Schultz O (2000) Matrix-mixed culture: New methodology for chondrocyte culture and preparation of cartilage transplants. J Biomed Mater Res 49:305–311

6. Spitzer RS, Perka C, Lindenhayn K (1999) In vitro cultivation of rabbit and porcine periosteal cells in matrix-mixed culture for bone replacement. International Meeting of the SIROT, April 16–19, 1999, Sydney, Australia, SIROT 296–300

7. Stern S, Lindenhayn K, Schultz O, Perka C (2000) The cultivation of porcine cells from the nucleus pulposus in a fibrin/hyaluronic acid matrix. Acta Orthop Scand 71:496–502

8. Stern S, Lindenhayn K, Perka C (2002) Human intervertebral disc cell culture for disc disorders (submitted)

CHAPTER 18

Chondrocytes and Collagen Gels 18

ULRICH SCHNEIDER and KARSTEN GAVÉNIS

Introduction

Since Hunter's observation in 1743, that cartilage "once destroyed, is not repaired", numerous techniques have been developed to treat cartilage defects. The poor self-healing capacity of cartilage limits the existing procedures. Regenerated tissue is only cartilage-like, with different biochemical and biomechanical characteristics in contrast to the surrounding cartilage and a more or less poor bonding. In recent years, Brittberg's method of the transplantation of autologous chondrocytes [3, 8] in suspension has been improved by the use of different carriers. Among these scaffolds, including agarose, alginate, matrices of polylactic acid, meshes of different collagens and many others [1, 2, 4, 7, 10–12], collagen gels are of particular value [5, 6, 9, 13–16]. They are biodegradable, they cause a very limited, if any inflammatory reaction, and offer a three-dimensional surrounding, which is similar to that of hyaline cartilage. Collagen gels are able to take any shape desired and therefore adapt to any defect size. In contrast to meshes or fleece, where cells are only seeded onto the surface, chondrocytes in gels show an even distribution, which allows a homogeneous synthesis of matrix components.

In this study, we compared several collagen type I gel systems with respect to handling, biomechanical and biochemical characteristics under *in vitro* and *in vivo* conditions.

Materials and Methods

Human articular cartilage samples from patients undergoing knee arthoplasty were digested with 1 mg/mL collagenase B. The released chondrocytes were seeded in a 10 cm culture dish and cultured until passage 2 in DMEM medium containing 10% FBS.

Released chondrocytes were cultured in 3 different collagen type I systems. Nine volumes collagen type I from calf skin (3% sterile aqueous solution, Roche Diagnostics, Indianapolis, USA) were mixed with 1 volume 10 × DMEM. One volume collagen type I from rat tail (ARS Arthro AG, Esslingen, Germany) was mixed with 1 volume 2 × DMEM/2 M HEPES (0.93:0.07). Eight volumes Atelocollagen (3% aqueous solution, Koken, Tokyo, Japan) were given to 1 volume 0.05 N NaOH/2.2% $NaHCO_3$/200 mM HEPES solution and 1 volume 10 × Ham's F-12. The collagen solutions were suspended with chondrocytes in a final concentration of 1×10^6 cells/mL. They were allowed to gel in 24 well plates with 1 mL in each well, overlaid with DMEM medium and cultured under standard conditions (37 °C and 5% CO_2) in a humidified incubator for up to 4 weeks. For all matrices, weight was determined before and after cultivation. Subsequently, matrices were subject to mechanical testing and analyzed.

After cultivation, matrices were fixed overnight in a phosphate-buffered solution of 4% para-formaldehyde and embedded in paraffin. Five μm sections were stained with hematoxylineosin, toluidine blue and safranin-O according to standard protocols. Images were captured by a Leica microscope and prepared using the Discus software.

Cross-sectioned slices were incubated with a polyclonal antibody to human collagen type II (Biotrend, Köln, Germany). Staining was visualized using the streptavidin/biotin technique (Vectastain ABC Kit, Vector Laboratories, Burlingame, U.S.A.). Diaminobenzidine (DAB Peroxidase Substrate Kit, Vector Laboratories, Burlingame, U.S.A.) was used as the developing substrate. The specifity of the immunoperoxidase staining was verified by omission of the primary antibody and the use of matrices without cells.

Cell viability was tested by TUNEL staining of apoptotic cells (Promega, Madison, USA), while proliferation was visualized by immunochemical staining of Ki-67, a protein specific for proliferating cells, according to the manufacturer's protocol (NeoMarkers, Fremont, USA).

Mechanical properties of the matrix samples were determined by an unconfined compression creep test. A constant force of 10 mN was applied by a mechanical testing device (Zwick, Ulm, Germany) uniaxially for 30 seconds on the matrix. The distance was determined with respect to the time and the thickness of the matrix. Finally, the applied force was removed and the retardation of the matrix was monitored for 30 seconds.

For the *in vivo* assay, matrix samples of the different collagen gels were loaded with passage 2 or freshly prepared chondrocytes and implanted subcutaneous in nude mice (BALB/c-nu/nu). The mice were sacrifices after 3 months. Recovered samples were fixed in formalin, and histological and immunohistochemical staining was performed as described.

Results and Discussion

The general appearance of the 3 tested collagen type I gel systems was quiet similar. The viscosity of the gels was generally moderate. They could be easily and homogenously mixed with the suspended chondrocytes and porn into different wells as desired. After gelling, samples of all 3 matrix systems could be easily handled with forceps. So all 3 investigated systems had the general advantages of collagen gels. Nevertheless, the 3 systems revealed significant differences, which might influence the clinical use. In the course of cultivation, a loss of weight occurred concerning all three gel systems, which in the case of Roche collagen type I was so significant, that the intrinsic stability of the samples was lost. After 1 week of culture, the Roche samples broke in pieces and we were not able to handle them. This loss of weight, which in the case of Roche collagen led to a breakdown of stability, might be due to an enhanced production of matrix metalloproteases or other catabolic enzymes. Generally, catabolic processes seem to exceed anabolic processes of ECM production under *in vitro* conditions.

The observed loss of sample weight seems not to be a characteristic of collagen gels in general, because it is dependent of the cell number included in the gel.

As a consequence of mechanical failure, Roche collagen had to be excluded from the study. Both Atelocollagen and Ars Arthro collagen revealed good mechanical stability. Figure 18.1 shows the mechanical characteristics of Atelocollagen and Ars Arthro collagen with respect to creeping abilities and retardation.

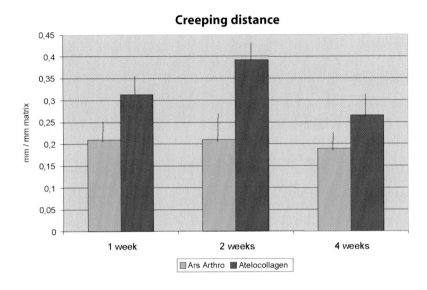

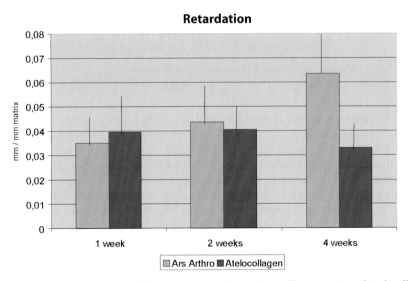

Fig. 18.1. Creeping and retardation distances of Ars Arthro collagen type I and Atelocollagen.

HE x20   Collagen Type II x63

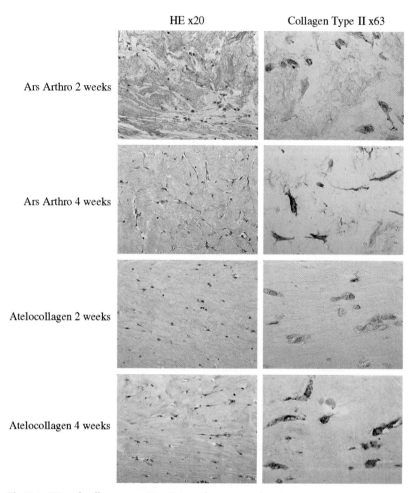

Fig 18.2. HE and collagen type II staining of passage 2 chondrocytes.

One of the main advantages of gels in comparison to other matrix systems is shown in Fig. 18.2. Both Atelocollagen and Ars Arthro collagen revealed a homogeneous distribution of cells throughout the course of culture. Cell number increased only slightly, which is consistent with results we obtained from a proliferation assay. This assay (immunochemical detection of Ki-67, a protein specific for proliferating cells) only stained very few chondrocytes. Possibly, cells in these three-dimensional gels were restricted in proliferation because they enclosed themselves by newly produced ECM. Collagen type II could be stained in both gel systems to a nearly equivalent amount. It was synthesized early in cultivation and persisted until the end of the investigated time period. Collagen type II was stored mainly in the pericellular region and did not built a territorial matrix, characteristic for hyaline cartilage. Quantitative PCR showed a collagen type II gene expression only in the beginning of the culture and only in small amounts. Catabolic effects, which might be responsible for the loss of weight did not affect the newly synthesized collagen type II.

Although, there was a distinct production of collagen type II detectable under *in vitro* conditions, both intensity and distribution was far from the situation in normal hyaline cartilage. To improve culture conditions, we introduced 2 major changes. First, after gelling, Atelocollagen and Ars Arthro collagen were implanted subcutanously in nude mice. Second, in addition to passage 2 cells, we used freshly prepared chondrocytes. The nude mouse systems offers the advantage of a cultivation system, which is much closer to the *in vivo* situation. The use of freshly prepared cells minimizes any de-differentiation, which takes place as soon as chondrocytes are seeded in monolayer. These two changes lead to striking improvements (Fig. 18.3). Compared to cultured chondrocytes *in vitro*, introducing the matrices in nude mice generally enhanced collagen type II production. The production and especially distribution of collagen type II was even better when freshly prepared cells were used. Cells immediately started to build an ECM, which with respect to collagen type II strongly resembled hyaline cartilage.

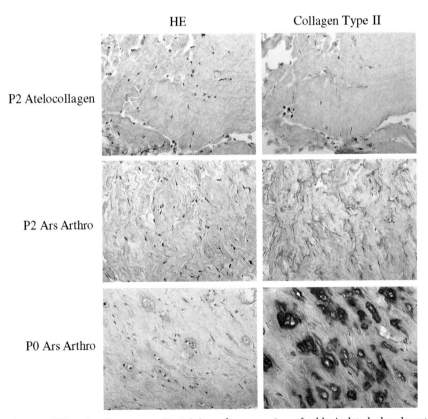

Fig 18.3. HE and collagen type II staining of passage 2 or freshly isolated chondrocytes 3 weeks after subcutaneous implantation in the nude mice.

Summary

In summary, the presented study shows the advantages of collagen gels, especially in combination with *in vivo* culture systems. Nevertheless, the investigated collagen type I gel systems showed these advantages to a different degree. While all collagen gels lost weight to some extend, the Roche collagen type I, which lacks clinical approval, lost its intrinsic cohesion. After one week, it had to be excluded from the experiments. In contrast, Ars Arthro collagen type I and Atelocollagen were easy to handle and showed good mechanical characteristics, although Ars Arthro collagen I had a slightly better outcome, with respect to retardation. The Atelocollagen samples were slightly varying in viscosity. This inconsistency of quality might be due to the fact, that Atelocollagen is a side product of cattle not raised exclusively for Atelocollagen production. The bovine origin of Atelocollagen might be a problem for clinical application in general. Ars Arthro collagen type I, which is gained from tails of inbreeding rats offers a controlled quality.

Experiments performed with Göttinger mini pigs showed an excellent bonding when artificial knee defects where filled with this matrix. Currently, a clinical trial with Ars Arthro collagen type I is going on, which has to prove if this technique of cartilage cell transplantation is suitable for clinical application (Fig. 18.4).

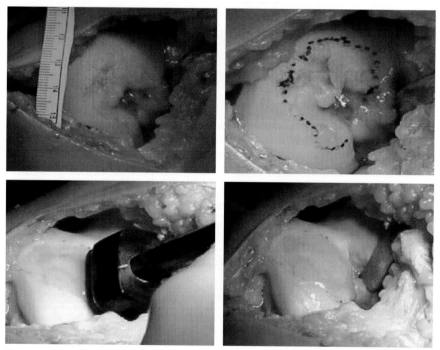

Fig 18.4. Ars Arthro collagen type I matrix seeded with autologeous chondrocytes and filled in a cartilage knee defect.

References

1. Behrens P, Ehlers EM, Kochermann KU, Rohwedel J, Russlies M, Plotz W (1999) Neues Ther-apieverfahren für lokalisierte Knorpeldefekte –Ermutigende Resultate mit der autologen Chondrozytenimplantation. MMW Fortschr Med 141:49–51
2. Ben-Yishay A, Grande DA, Menche SS (1992) Repair of articular cartilage defects using col-lagen-chondrocyte allografts. Trans Orthop Res Society 17:174
3. Brittberg M, Lindahl A, Nilsson A, Ohlsson C, Isaksson O, Peterson L (1994) Treatment of deep cartilage defects in the knee with autologous chondrocyte transplantation. N Engl J Med 331:889–895
4. Frenkel SR, Toolan B, Menche D, Pitman MI, Pachence JM (1997) Chondrocyte transplanta-tion using a collagen bilayer matrix for cartilage repair. J Bone Joint Surg-Br 79:831–836
5. Katsube K, Ochi M, Uchio Y, Maniwa S, Matsusaki M, Tobita M, Iwasa J (2000) Repair of artic-ular cartilage defects with cultured chondrocytes in Atelocollagen gel. Comparison with cul-tured chondrocytes in suspension. Arch Orthop Trauma Surg 120:121–127
6. Kawamura S, Wakitani S, Kimura T, Maeda A, Caplan AI, Shino K, Ochi T (1998) Articular cartilage repair. Rabbit experiments with a collagen gel-biomatrix and chondrocytes cul-tured in it. Acta Orthop Scand 69:56–62
7. Nehrer S, Breinan HA, Ramappa A et al. (1998) Chondrocyte-seeded collagen matrices implanted in a chondral defect in a canine model. Biomaterials 19:2313–2328
8. Peterson L, Minas T, Brittberg M, Nilsson A, Sjogren-Jansson E, Lindahl A (2000) Two- to 9-year outcome after autologous chondrocyte transplantation of the knee. Clin Orthop 374:212–234
9. Schuman L, Buma P, Versleyen D, de Man B, van der Kraan PM, van den Berg WB, Hommin-ga GN (1995) Chondrocyte behaviour within different types of collagen gel in vitro. Bioma-terials 16:809–814
10. Sohn DH, Lottman LM, Lum LY, Kim SG, Pedowitz RA, Coutts RD, Sah RL (2002) Effect of grav-ity on localization of chondrocytes implanted in cartilage defects. Clin Orthop 394:254–262
11. Solchaga LA, Goldberg VM, Caplan AI (2001) Cartilage regeneration using principles of tis-sue engineering. Clin Orthop 391 [Suppl]:S161–170
12. Speer DP, Chvapil M, Volz RG, Holmes MD (1979) Enhancement of healing in osteochondral defects by collagen sponge implants. Clin Orthop 144:326–335
13. Uchio Y, Ochi M, Matsusaki M, Kurioka H, Katsube K (2000) Human chondrocyte prolifera-tion and matrix synthesis cultured in Atelocollagen gel. J Biomed Mater Res 50:138–143
14. van Susante JL, Buma P, van Osch GJ, Versleyen D, van der Kraan PM, van der Berg WB, Hom-minga GN (1995) Culture of chondrocytes in alginate and collagen carrier gels. Acta Orthop Scand 66:549–556.
15. Wakitani S, Kimura T, Hirooka A, Ochi T, Yoneda M, Yasui N, Owaki H, Ono K (1989) Repair of rabbit articular surfaces with allograft chondrocytes embedded in collagen gel. J Bone Joint Surg-Br 71:74–80.
16. Yasui N, Osawa S, Ochi T, Nakashima H, Ono K (1982) Primary culture of chondrocytes embedded in collagen gels. Exp Cell Biol 50:92–100

CHAPTER 19

Fabrication of Cartilage-Polymer Constructs 19 for Articular Cartilage Repair

ULRICH NÖTH, ARNE BERNER, RICHARD TULI, ACHIM BATTMANN, CHRISTIAN HENDRICH, JOCHEN EULERT and ROCKY S. TUAN

Introduction

There are a number of treatment strategies for the repair of articular cartilage defects that are currently in clinical use or at the experimental stage of development. Treatment strategies currently in clinical use are lavage and debridement, abrasion chondroplasty, microfracture techniques, subchondral drilling, transplantation of periosteal or perichondrial grafts, transplantation of osteochondral autografts or allografts, and autologous chondrocyte transplantation [1–4, 7, 8, 14, 15, 23]. Techniques currently at an experimental stage include the implantation of biocompatible matrices (e.g. agarose, alginate, collagen gels or sponges, hyaluronic acid, polylactic- or polyglycolic acid) alone or in combination with chondrocytes or growth factors, such as members of the transforming growth factor superfamily-β (TGF-β) [10– 12, 16, 18, 19, 22, 26, 27]. Transplantation of cell populations, such as marrow-derived mesenchymal stem cells (mMSCs) or periosteal cells that are capable of differentiation into chondrocytes, and genetic engineering with the use of cells as a platform for delivery of gene products or retroviral transduction of genes, are considered promising techniques to enhance articular cartilage repair [9, 17, 21]. We have describe a new experimental approach for *in vitro* cartilage tissue engineering consisting of cell-polymer constructs formed by press-coating bioresorbable polymer with pellet cell cultures of mMSCs [20].

Polymer-Coating Technique

Marrow-derived MSCs were isolated from the femoral head of patients diagnosed with osteoarthritis and undergoing total hip arthroplasty, as previously described [13, 20]. D,D-L,L-poly-lactic acid polymer blocks (OPLA®, Kensey Nash Corp., Exton, PA) were used for the coating procedure. The blocks have an apparent density of 0.0900 (+/– 0.0050), void volumes of 90 to 92% (measured by helium pycnometry) of their apparent volumes, and molecular weights of 100,000 to 135,000 kDa after commercial gamma sterilization [5, 6]. The rate of biodegradation of the polymer is governed by multiple variables of the local tissues or culture environments. In most mammalian connective tissues OPLA® is hydrolyzed to microscopic fragments by 6 to 9 months and completely metabolized out of the tissue by 12 months post implantation, with faster hydrolysis in the presence of osteoinductive morphogens [5, 6].

Culture-expanded
MSCs

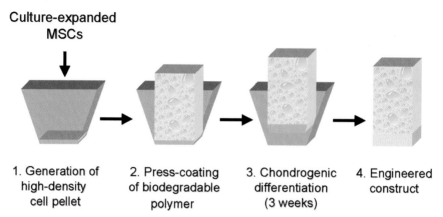

1. Generation of high-density cell pellet

2. Press-coating of biodegradable polymer

3. Chondrogenic differentiation (3 weeks)

4. Engineered construct

Fig. 19.1. Illustration of the press-coating technique. A biodegradable polymer block is press-coated with hMSCs and cultured in a chondrogenic differentiation medium over a three week time period.

The polymer press-coating technique is shown in Fig. 19.1 [20]. High-density pellet cell cultures were initiated from 1.5×10^6 mMSCs in 50 mL conical tubes by centrifugation ($500 \times g$ for 5 min), and formed cell pellets of 5 mm in diameter and 2 mm in thickness at the bottom of the tubes. The medium was removed and a polymer block was gently pressed onto each high-density cell pellet. To prevent the polymer from floating, the cell-polymer constructs were cultured initially in a minimal (300 µl) volume of serum-free, chemically defined chondrogenic differentiation medium supplemented with 10 ng/mL TGF-β1. After attachment of the cell pellet to the polymer surface was assured (after 3 to 4 hours) 2.7 mL of medium was added. The floating constructs coated with mMSCs were incubated for 3 weeks at 37°C in 5% CO_2. At the time of harvest translucent cartilage-like layers were seen forming on top of the polymers along the originally coated surface (Fig. 19.2). The layers appeared to be about 0.1 to 0.15 cm thick, without interruption along the surface, but extended to different depths into the polymer, depending on the surface structure of the polymer [20].

In Vitro Analysis

Histochemical and immunohistochemical analysis of the cell-polymer constructs maintained in the chondrogenic differentiation medium for 3 weeks and stained with HE showed morphologically distinct, round chondrocyte-like cells embedded in extracellular matrix. Staining with alcian blue revealed the presence of a negatively charged sulfated proteoglycan-rich extracellular matrix [20]. Immunostaining of the cell-polymer sections detected the presence of collagen type II (Fig. 19.3). Collagen type I staining was highest at the outer perichondrium-like surface and the surfaces facing the polymer embedded in the cartilage layer [20].

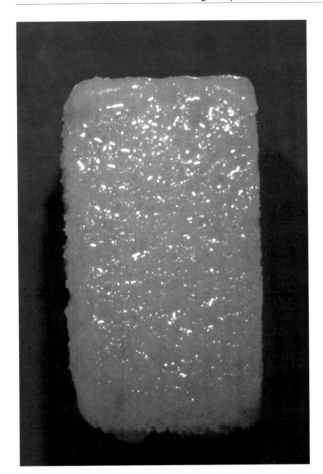

Fig. 19.2.
Micrograph of a cell-polymer construct consisting of a 1×0.5×0.5 cm polymer block coated with $1.5×10^6$ mhMSCs. Note the translucent cartilage layer, which has formed on top of the polymer.

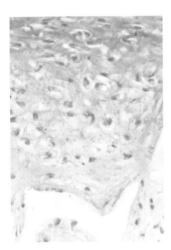

Fig. 19.3.
Immunohistochemical analysis of the engineered cartilage layer showing chondrocyte-like cells embedded in a collagen type II-rich extracellular matrix.

Total RNA was isolated from the cartilage layer bonded to the polymer after 3 weeks of culture. RT-PCR analysis revealed the mRNA expression of the chondrogenic marker genes collagen types II, IX, X, XI, and aggrecan by the engineered constructs (Fig. 19.4). Expression of collagen type I was also found [20]. The gene expression profile resembled that of positive control cell pellets cultured without polymer. Cartilage constructs and positive control cell pellets generated from the different donors showed the same gene expression pattern.

Preliminary in Vivo Results

Nude rats (rnu[H] rats) obtained from Dr. Hedrich (Institut für Versuchstierkunde, Medizinische Hochschule Hannover, Germany) were used as an *in vivo* model [24, 25]. Animals at an age between 3 and 6 months were narcotized by an Isoflurane® anesthesia. An osteochondral defect of 1.5 mm in diameter and 5 mm in depth was drilled into the trochlear groove using a crown trephine (Meisinger, Düsseldorf, Germany). The *in vitro* fabricated polymer-cartilage constructs were implanted into the defect in a press-fit manner. Immediately after surgery the animals showed an unrestricted activity. The animals were sacrificed after 4 weeks and specimens were obtained for histochemical analysis. Staining with HE showed an excellent bonding of the implanted cartilage layer to the surrounding cartilage. Also, beginning of bone formation was seen in the remaining volume of the PLA-polymer underneath the cartilage layer (Fig. 19.5). Currently, more detailed histochemical and immunohistochemical analysis of the matrix composition of the engineered cartilage layer after 3 and 6 months are performed.

Conclusion

We have developed a new technique for *in vitro* engineering of cartilage by press-coating biodegradable polymer with mMSCs that show promise for the reconstruction of articular cartilage defects. The technique involves the utilization of mMSCs prepared as

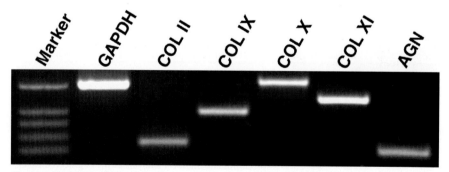

Fig. 19.4. RT-PCR analysis of the *in vitro* engineered cartilage constructs showing collagen type II, IX, X, XI, and aggrecan expression.

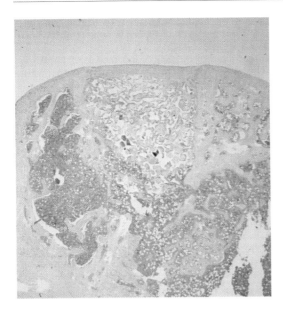

Fig. 19.5.
Histochemical analysis (HE staining) of a cartilage-polymer construct implanted in the rat trochlea after 4 weeks. Note that the implanted cartilage layer is well integrated into the surrounding cartilage.

high-density pellet cell cultures that are subsequently press-coated onto the surface of porous biodegradable polymer blocks. Our immunohistochemical analysis of sections of the engineered cartilage construct detected collagen type I predominantly at the surface of the construct and the surfaces facing the polymer embedded in the cartilage layer, suggesting the formation of fibrous, perichondrium-like layers at these regions. Because type I collagen was found within the cartilage layer, the phenotype of the engineered cartilage cannot be strictly defined as articular cartilage. Nevertheless, type II collagen, a typical marker of hyaline cartilage could be detected histochemically and by RT-PCR. First animal studies have shown promising results with good integration of the engineered cartilage layer into the surrounding cartilage. Prior to implantation, the remaining volume of the polymer scaffold may be loaded with mMSCs and/or osteoinductive growth factors (e.g. BMP-2) to elicit osteogenesis *in situ* and enhance osseointegration of the construct. Furthermore, we propose that the press-coating technique might be useful in designing whole parts of a joint, such as the femoral condyle.

References

1. Baumgaertner MR, Cannon WD Jr, Vittori JM, Schmidt ES, Maurer RC (1990) Arthroscopic debridement of the arthritic knee. Clin Orthop 253:197–202
2. Bentley G (1992) Articular tissue grafts. Ann Rheum Dis 51:292–296
3. Bert JM, Maschka K (1989) The arthroscopic treatment of unicompartimental gonarthrosis: A five-year follow-up study of abrasion arthroplasty plus arthroscopic debridement and arthroscopic debridement alone. Arthroscopy 5:25–32
4. Bobic V (1996) Arthroscopic osteochondral autograft transplantation in anterior cruciate ligament reconstruction: A preliminary clinical study. Knee Surg Sports Traumatol Arthroscopy 3:262–264

5. Brekke JH (1996) A rationale for delivery of osteoinductive proteins. Tissue Eng 2:97–106
6. Brekke JH, Toth JM (1998) Principles of tissue engineering applied to programmable osteogenesis. J Biomed Mater Res (Appl Biomater) 43:380–398
7. Brittberg M (1999) Autologous chondrocyte transplantation. Clin Orthop 367:147–155
8. Buckwalter JA, Lohmander S (1994) Operative treatment of osteoarthrosis. Current practice and future development. J Bone Joint Surg-A 76:1405–1418
9. Evans CH, Ghivizzani SC, Smith P, Shuler FD, Mi Z, Robins PD (2000) Using gene therapy to protect and restore cartilage. Clin Orthop 379 [Suppl]:214–219
10. Fortier LA, Lust G, Nixon AJ (1999) Insulin-like growth factor-I enhances cell-based articular cartilage resurfacing. Trans Orthop Res Soc 45:58
11. Freed LE, Grande DA, Lingbin Z, Emmanual J, Marquis JC, Langer R (1994) Joint resurfacing using allograft chondrocytes and synthetic polymer scaffolds. J Biomed Mater Res 28:891–899
12. Frenkel SR, Toolan B, Menche D, Pitman MI, Pachence JM (1997) Chondrocyte transplantation using a collagen bilayer matrix for cartilage repair. J Bone Joint Surg-Br 79:831–836
13. Haynesworth SE, Goshima J, Goldberg VM, Caplan AI (1992) Characterization of cells with osteogenic potential from human marrow. Bone 13:81–88
14. Hoikka VE, Jaroma HJ, Ritsila VA (1990) Reconstruction of the patella articulation with periostal grafts. 4-year follow-up of 13 cases. Acta Orthop Scand 61:36–39
15. Homminga GN, Bulstra SK, Bouwmeester PS, van der Linden AJ (1990) Perichondral grafting of cartilage lesions of the knee. J Bone Joint Surg-Br 72:1003–1007
16. Hunziker EB, Rosenberg LC (1996) Repair of partial-thickness articular cartilage defects. Cell recruitment from the synovium. J Bone Joint Surg-A 78:721–733
17. Johnstone BJ, Yoo U (1999) Autologous mesenchymal progenitor cells in articular cartilage repair. Clin Orthop (abstract) 367:156
18. Martin JA, Buckwalter JA (1996) Articular cartilage aging and degeneration. Sports Med Arthroscop Rev 4:263–269
19. Nehrer S, Breinan HA, Ashkar S, Shortkroff S, Minas T, Sledge CB, Yannas IV, Spector M (1998) Characteristics of articular chondrocytes seeded in collagen matrices *in vitro*. Tissue Eng 4:175–184
20. Nöth U, Tuli R, Osyczka AM, Danielson KG, Tuan RS (2002) In vitro engineered cartilage constructs produced by press-coating biodegradable polymer with human mesenchymal stem cells. Tissue Eng 8:131–143
21. O'Driscoll SW (1999) Articular cartilage regeneration using periosteum. Clin Orthop 367 [Suppl]:186–203
22. Rahford B, Weisser J, Sternkopf F, Aigner T, von der Mark K, Brauer R (1998) Transplantation of allograft chondrocytes embedded in agarose gel into cartilage defects of rabbits. Osteoarthritis Cartilage 6:50–65
23. Rodrigo JJ, Stadman JR, Silliman JF, Fulstone HA (1994) Improvement of full-thickness chondral defect healing in the human knee after debridement and microfracture using continuous passive motion. Am J Knee Surg 7:109–115
24. Schuurman HJ (1995) The nude rat. Hum Exp Toxicol 14:122–125
25. Schwinzer R, Hedrich HJ, Wonigeit K (1989) T cell differentiation in athymic nude rats (rnu/rnu): demonstration of a distorted T cell subset structure by flow cytometry analysis. Eur J Immunol 19:1841–1847
26. Solchaga LA, Lundberg M, Yoo JU, Huibregtse BA, Goldberg VM, Caplan AI (1999) Hyaluronic acid-based polymers in the treatment of osteochondral defects. Trans Orthop Res Soc 45:56
27. Vacanti CA, Langer R, Schloo B, Vacanti JP (1991) Synthetic polymers seeded with chondrocytes provide a template for new cartilage formation. Plast Reconstr Surg 88:753–759

Differentiation of Human and Murine Chondrogenic Cells Encapsulated in Ultra-High Viscosity Alginate*

20

CHRISTIAN HENDRICH, MEIKE WEBER, ACHIM BATTMANN, NORBERT SCHÜTZE,
CONRAD JULIUS, ANDRE STEINERT, MANUELA FALTIN, SABINE BALLING,
HEIKO ZIMMERMANN, ULRICH NÖTH and ULRICH ZIMMERMANN

Introduction

Transplantation of autologous chondrocytes cultured and expanded under *in vitro* conditions has yielded good to excellent long-term results in 92% of circumscript femoral cartilage lesions (see chapter 1) [22]. A major problem of chondrocyte expansion is the phenomenon of de-differentiation after multiple cell passages [21]. When cultured in monolayers, chondrocytes change their appearance to a fibroblast-like morphology and switch from production of hyaline cartilage-specific collagen type II (and chondroitin-6-sulfate) to synthesis of collagen type I [6, 33]. Re-differentiation and formation of hyaline components can be achieved by encapsulation of the cells in a three-dimensional matrix [15, 20]. Alginate has been extensively employed for *in vitro* cultures and in animal studies for articular cartilage repair [11, 19, 20, 35]. However, as outlined in Zimmermann et al. (chapter 9, this issue), commercial alginates provoke foreign body reactions, especially when implanted in rats exhibiting an elevated macrophage system. Immunoreactive alginates will not receive medical approval because they do not meet the demands of the guidelines of the American Society for Testing and Materials (ASTM) and GMP/ISO 9000 [9]. Use of commercial alginates for *in vitro* and animal studies is also not recommendable because the contaminants might affect the metabolic, secretory and/or growth properties of the entrapped cells in an unpredictable way.

In contrast, ultra-high viscosity (UHV) alginates extracted from bacteria-free stipes of brown algae and purified with the removal of mitogenic, cytotoxic and apoptosis-inducing impurities is of clinical grade (CG) and thus completely biocompatible (see chapter 9). *In vitro* and *in vivo* studies with Langerhans's islets and parathyroid allogenic tissue segments encapsulated in UHV/CG-alginate have demonstrated (Bohrer et al., unpublished results) [26] that insulin secretion and parathormone release are not affected, provided that the alginate concentration is properly adjusted. This work has also shown (see chapter 9) that the cross-linking procedure with diva-

* We are very grateful to M. Behringer, P. Geßner and A. Steinbach for skilful technical assistance. This work was supported by grants from the Landesgewerbeanstalt (High-Tech-Offensive des Freistaates Bayern), from the Deutsche Forschungsgemeinschaft (Zi 99/16–1) and BMBF (VDI 16SV1329) to U. Z., by grants from the Deutsche Forschungsgemeinschaft (He 2460/4–1) to C. H. and by a grant from BMBF (VDI 16SV1366/0) to H. Z.

lent cations is also important. These observations have obvious implications for the development of UHV/CG-alginate-based encapsulation procedures of single chondrocytes and other cells undergoing chondrogenesis. An understanding of how the extracellular matrix affects the viability and secretory profiles of entrapped cells is crucial for developing tissue engineered constructs for cartilage repair.

In this chapter we report on the chondrogenic differentiation of UHV/CG-alginate encapsulated human chondrocytes, human mesenchymal stem cells (MSCs) as well as on C3H10T1/2, a mouse mesenchymal stem cell line stably transfected with bone morphogenetic protein-4 (BMP-4 cells). MSCs and BMP-4 cells can be amplified without limitation (unlike chondrocytes) and they undergo chondrogenesis, when immobilized and cultured in a favorable environment. Data obtained *in vitro* and *in vivo* indicate that UHV/CG-alginate meets the demands for an optimal tissue engineering matrix, for which medical approval can be granted. Interestingly, the results also revealed differences in the histological appearance and the production of cartilage-specific matrix components between the three cell types. The different responses were more cell-specific than matrix-specific. This finding is critical to the current discussion on proposed therapies for articular cartilage lesions, which try to circumvent the shortage of autologous chondrocytes by transplanting MSCs or genetically engineered cells.

Murine BMP-4 Transfected C3H10T1/2 Cells

Puromycin-resistant C3H10T1/2 cells, stably transfected with BMP-4 were established by Ahrens et al. [1]. Proliferation and differentiation were studied under monolayer (2D-) and encapsulation (3D-) conditions (for details, see [33]). The cells were cultured in complete growth medium (containing 5 µg/mL puromycin). After 3 days, when the cells were nearly confluent, the growth medium was replaced by differentiation medium. This medium consisted of complete growth medium containing β-glycerophosphate (10 mM) and ascorbic acid (50 µg/mL).

When cultured in monolayer over 17 days the cells assumed a fibroblast-like morphology, even after addition of differentiation medium. Proliferation was moderate. On day 17 the cell number has increased by a factor of 3 to 4. Throughout the experimental period the level of alkaline phosphatase (ALP; an osteogenic marker) remained low (about 1.5 to 2.5 pg/min/mg/cell protein), as determined by measuring the release of p-nitrophenol from p-nitrophenylphosphate [7, 13]. Immunohistological analysis performed on day 17 revealed an intense reactivity for collagen type I (a marker for de-differentiated chondrocytes), but only a weak reaction for collagen type II. Chondroitin-4-sulfate (a component of hyaline cartilage but also found in other tissues) and chondroitin-6-sulfate (a marker for hyaline cartilage) could not be detected. Consistent with this real time quantitative RT-PCR [10] yielded very low levels of collagen type II mRNA [33].

Opposite results were obtained when the adherent cells were detached (0.1% trypsin/EDTA) and encapsulated (seeding suspension density 1×10^6 cells per mL) by cross-linking a 0.5% w/v UHV/CG-alginate solution (extracted from *Laminaria pallida*) with external 20 mM Ca^{2+} (see chapter 9). Micro-encapsulation suppressed proliferation and the cells became spherical and immediately up-regulated type II collagen mRNA as revealed by real time RT-PCR (Fig. 20.1). Although this up-regulation was followed by a down-regulation on day 6, mRNA level increased continuously with ongoing culture after day 10. Encapsulated cells were also characterized by an up-regulation of collagen type I mRNA with the peak value on day 10. The following decrease in mRNA coincided with the second up-regulation phase of type II collagen mRNA (see Fig. 20.1). Type X collagen mRNA, a marker for hypertrophic chondrogenesis [3, 5, 32], could not be detected [29]. The osteogenic marker Cbfa-1 was also not up-regulated [29]. However, in encapsulated BMP-4 cells, the osteogenic marker ALP showed a very pronounced and transient up-regulation. A detectable increase in ALP activity was usually observed on day 6. Immunostaining performed on various days of culture confirmed the real time RT-PCR results. On day 17 the central cells and cell clusters were encircled completely by dense depositions of type II collagen. These areas also exhibited positive reactivity with chondroitin-6-sulfate antibodies. Chondroitin-4-sulfate was also found, but there was only very weak staining for type X collagen (see Table 20.1).

Similar *in vitro* results were found for BMP-4 cells when the encapsulation was performed with 1% w/v UHV/CG-alginate, and when Ba^{2+} ions were used instead of Ca^{2+} ions for external gelling. Production of type II collagen matrix proteins was also found when the BMP-4 cells were entrapped in an alginate matrix (0.5% w/v), homoge-

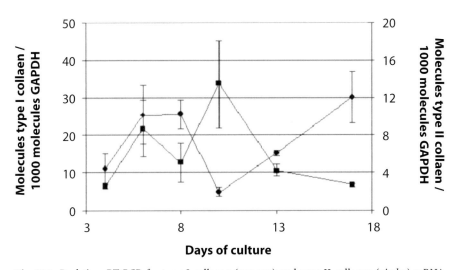

Days of culture

Fig. 20.1. Real time RT-PCR for type I collagen (*squares*) and type II collagen (*circles*) mRNA expression in murine BMP-4 transfected C3H10T1/2 cells encapsulated in alginate microcapsules. Encapsulation was performed using a 0.5% (w/v) UHV/CG-alginate solution that was cross-linked with 20 mM Ca^{2+}. On Day 3, the culture medium was replaced by differentiation medium. For relative quantification, the amount of target gene was normalized to the housekeeping gene GAPDH. Thus, the mRNA values are presented as numbers of molecules per 1000 molecules GAPDH. Data represent the mean $\pm$ SD of at least three independent experiments. For further details, see Weber et al. [33].

neously cross-linked by injection of $BaCl_2$ crystals into the alginate droplets (internal gelling; see chapter 9) [38].

In contrast to the *in vitro* data, only very weak chondrogenic differentiation of BMP-4 cells encapsulated in Ba^{2+} cross-linked alginate (1% w/v) was observed 4 weeks after transplantation into an osteochondral defect of athymic nude rats (rnu^H rats) [27, 28]. For transplantation, cylindrical transplants about 0.5 cm in lenhth were formed to fit into the defects. The grafts were kept in differentiation medium for 1 to 14 days before transplantation. Histological analysis of the retrieved transplants showed [29] that the defects were almost completely filled by the graft, even though some cysts as well as cracks in the alginate matrix could frequently be seen (even in control transplants consisting of alginate only). There was no evidence for synovitis, angiogenesis, ossification or formation of giant cells, at and around the transplantation site. Inflammatory reactions, i.e. invasion of the transplants by granulocytes and mononuclear cells was also not observed. Cells were viable as revealed by propidium iodide staining. More than 25% of the cells formed clusters. For quantification, the data were evaluated using the O'Driscoll score [17]. The O'Driscoll score was originally introduced for the evaluation of cartilage repairs at the surface of articular cartilage. In the experiments reported here, the main part of the transplant was located within the bone, i.e. the thickness of the cartilage layer of the joint represented only a small part of the entire osteochondral defect. Therefore, a modified O'Driscoll score comprising 13 points was used for transplant rating. As detailed in the legend to Fig. 20.2 the points were assigned to defect filling (maximum 4 points), structural integrity (maximum 4 points), cellularity (maximum 3 points), and cell clustering (maximum 2 points). The evaluation yielded 1.00 ± 0.82 (mean $\pm$ SD) points for the structural integrity, no points for cell clustering, 0.50 ± 1.00 for cellularity, and 3.50 ± 1.00 points for defect filling (see Fig. 20.2), thus resulting in an O'Driscoll score of 5.00 ± 2.16 (n = 4).

Evaluation of the corresponding immunostainings revealed low production of type II collagen (Fig. 20.3A) and chondroitin-6-sulfate, as well as of chrondroitin-4-sulfate and type X collagen, but moderate expression of type I collagen (Table 20.1). This indicates that the BMP-4 cells are apparently de-differentiated to a large extent after a transplantation period of 1 month.

Human Mesenchymal Stem Cells and Chondrocytes

Bone marrow-derived MSCs and chondrocytes were isolated from the femoral head of an 8-year old patient undergoing resection arthroplasty because of complete dislocation of the hip as a result of cerebral palsy. The use of surgical waste for research purposes was approved by the Ethics Committee of the University of Würzburg. Chondrocytes and MSCs were isolated as described elsewhere [16, 25] and cultured in complete growth medium. Seventy to 80% confluency was reached for MSCs after 10 to 14 days and for chondrocytes after about 3 weeks. The adherent cells were detached with 0.1% trypsin/EDTA and were encapsulated by using 1% w/v UHV/CG-alginate and 20 mM external Ba^{2+} (seeding density 5×10^6 cells/mL).

Screening experiments for 2D- and 3D-cultures under *in vitro* conditions yielded similar results, as in the case of BMP-4 cells. For *in vivo* studies the rnu^H rat model was used. Cylindrically shaped, 0.5 cm long grafts of MSCs or chondrocytes were trans-

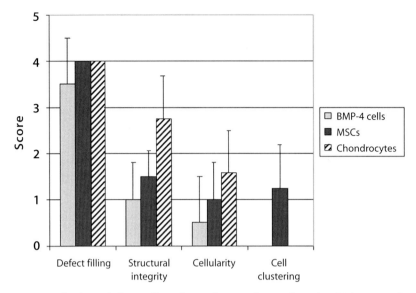

Fig. 20.2. Evaluation of the quality of 4-week transplants of murine BMP-4 transfected C3H10T1/2 cells (*grey columns*), human MSCs (*black columns*) and human chondrocytes (*dashed columns*), using a modified O'Driscoll score. Structural integrity (i), cell clustering (ii), cellularity (iii) and defect filling (iv), were assigned points: (i) normal = 4, beginning of a columnar organization = 3, no organization = 2, cyst or cracks = 1, severe disintegration = 0; (ii) no clusters = 2, <25% of the cells = 1, >25% of the cells = 0; (iii) normal = 3, moderate = 2, slight = 1 and none = 0; (iv) 111–125% = 3, 91–110% = 4, 76–90% = 3, 51–75% = 2, 26–50% = 1, <25% = 0. For further discussion, see text.

planted into osteochondral defects of similar size. Gross examination after 1 month showed an intact articular surface. In some samples a discrete depression was seen. Hematoxylin eosin (HE) staining revealed a complete filling of the defects and integration of the graft into the adjacent bone. Resorption of alginate was also not observed. The top of the cylindrical transplants was covered by a thin fibrocartilaginous layer of low cellularity. There was no evidence for synovitis and infection at and around the transplantation site in any of the 47 specimens investigated. The entrapped MSCs and chondrocytes were of spherical shape, they were viable and were partly organized in clusters. The number of cell clusters was higher for chondrocytes than for MSCs.

Calculations of the modified O'Driscoll score for chondrocytes (see Fig. 20.2) gave a value of 7.80 ± 2.28 (n = 5), 4.00 ± 0.00 points were assigned to defect filling, 2.75 ± 0.96 points to the structural integrity, 1.60 ± 0.89 points to cellularity and no points to cell clustering (because more than 25% of the cells were clustered, see above). The corresponding O'Driscoll score of the MSCs was calculated to be 7.75 ± 1.26 (n = 4). In this case, the points for defect filling, structural integrity, cellularity and cell clustering were 4.00 ± 0.00, 1.50 ± 0.58, 1.00 ± 0.82, and 1.25 ± 0.96, respectively (see Fig. 20.2).

Immunostaining revealed high production of collagen type II in the case of chondrocytes (Fig. 20.3B), but less for MSCs (Fig. 20.3C). Both cell types showed positive

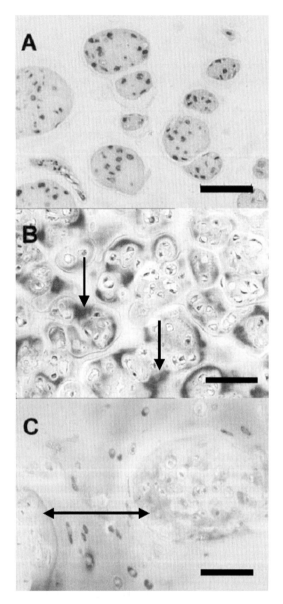

Fig. 20.3A–C.
Immunohistochemical staining on paraffin sections for type II collagen of encapsulated murine BMP-4 transfected C3H10T1/2 cells (**A**), human chondrocytes (**B**) and human MSCs (**C**). The grafts were transplanted in an osteo-chondral defect of the femoral trochlea of a rnuH nude rat. The joints were retrieved after 4 weeks for histological and immunohistological analysis [33]. Staining intensity was pronounced for chondrocytes (marked by *arrows*), but less of MSCs (marked by *double-headed arrows*). In contrast, BMP-4 cells showed very discrete indications for type II collagen production. Bar = 100 μm.

staining for chondroitin-6-sulfate, chondroitin-4-sulfate, and type I collagen. On average, the staining intensity was higher for chondrocytes than for MSCs. In contrast, the immunoreactivity for type X collagen was weak for both cell types. The findings summarized in Table 20.1 indicate that the chondrocytes, and to a lesser extent, the MSCs showed a chondrogenic re-differentiation after a transplantation period of 1 month.

Table 20.1. Immunoreactivity of different matrix markers for UHV/CG encapsulated murine BMP-4 transfected C3H10T1/2 mesenchymal progenitor cells, human MSCs and human chondrocytes

	BMP-4 cells *in vitro*[a,c]	BMP-4 cells *in vivo*[b,d]	MSCs *in vivo*[b,d]	Chondrocytes *in vivo*[b,d]
Collagen type I	+	++	++	++
Collagen type II	+++	+	+	+++
Chondroitin-4-sulphate	+++	+	++	++
Chondroitin-6-sulphate	++	+	++	++
Collagen type X	+	+	+	+

[a] The initial cell density was 1×10^6 cells/mL.
[b] The initial cell density was 5×10^6 cells/mL.
[c] Measurements were performed after 17 days in culture. Note that the alginate (0.5% w/v) was cross-linked with Ca^{2+}.
[d] Measurements were performed on 4-week transplants. Note that the alginate (1% w/v) was cross-linked with Ba^{2+}.
Key: + = detectable; ++ = moderate yield; +++ = intense yield.

Discussion

Grafts of encapsulated cells exhibiting chondrogenic differentiation must fulfill certain criteria for articular cartilage repair. The scaffold material must be biocompatible and should not have any adverse side effect on cell viability, metabolism, and secretory functions. It should prevent cells from floating out and cells such as macrophages from invading, at least during the phase of cartilage formation. The material must facilitate re-differentiation of *in vitro* expanded chondrogenic cells and long-term production of hyalinecartilage-specific matrix proteins. The initial mechanical properties of the scaffold material should allow surgical handling and allow the transplants to be shaped closely to the dimensions of the defect. In the long-term, the scaffold material must also be biodegradable without any immunological reactions to the degradation products.

These seminal conditions for a tissue engineered transplant designed for cartilage formation are largely fulfilled by UHV/CG-alginate scaffolds. This material can be produced reproducible on a large scale and is completely biocompatible, as shown by extensive animal studies including those in baboons (see chapter 9) [36]. This conclusion is also supported by the studies presented here. Athymic rnu[H] rats have a reduced immune system. Despite this, fibrosis and inflammatory reactions occurred upon implantation of commercial alginates [30] that contain significant amounts of mitogenic, cytotoxic, and apoptosis-inducing contaminants [14, 37]. Such reactions were not found for rnu[H] rats for any of the cells encapsulated.

A further advantage of UHV/CG-alginates is that the transplants can be very accurately fitted to the osteochondral defects even though the ultra-high viscosity poses problems in manufacture. Inspections of the sites 4 weeks after transplantation revealed that defect filling was (independent of the cell line encapsulated) quite excellent (see Fig. 20.2). Therefore, maximum points of the modified O'Driscoll score were assigned for this feature. However, transplants frequently showed a few cysts and cracks in the alginate matrix. The points for structural integrity in the O'Driscoll score were worse for BMP-4 cells (1.00) compared with MSCs (1.5) and particularly with chondrocytes (2.75). For controls, in which alginate was transplanted without cells, the corresponding value was 0.8, even lower than that for BMP-4 cells (unpublished data). These findings indicate that the extracellular matrix produced by the encapsulated cells contributes to the mechanical stability of the transplants. This effect is pronounced when type II collagen is produced at high concentrations, as in the case of chondrocytes (see above).

The mechanical stability of the alginate matrix, especially against shearing forces, can be increased in future experiments if the cross-linking process is improved. Mechanical stability depends on the viscosity and concentration of the alginate and on the choice of cross-linking divalent cations, but further optimization of these parameters is obviously not possible. As shown elsewhere [36, 37] the mechanical strength of matrices made from 1% UHV/CG-alginate and cross-linked with Ba^{2+} is significantly higher than that of matrices of low-viscosity (commercial) alginates of various concentrations cross-linked either with Ba^{2+} or other polyvalent cations. However (as outlined by Zimmermann et al., chapter 9), the crystal gun method significantly delays or prevents the formation of cysts, cracks and the subsequent disintegration of alginate transplants, as injecting $BaCl_2$ crystals improves cross-linking within the core of the alginate matrix. The crystals do not interfere with cell viability and production of hyalinecartilage-specific proteins as has been demonstrated by *in vitro* studies with BMP-4 cells [38]. Thus, this technique is a promising option for solving the problems of shear force instability in alginate matrices designed especially for cartilage repair. This technique also allows fine regulation of the onset and rate of degradation of the alginate matrix by controlling the number of injected crystals. This is important because the alginate matrix must be degradable once it has served its purpose in order to provide space for the growing tissue. Of equal importance is that the degradation of polymeric alginate chains leads ultimately to the release of the two monomers, mannuronic and guluronic acid, which are incorporated in enzymatic pathways for further degradation [2, 12, 19]. These authors did not report associated inflammatory reactions.

Cellularity, cell clustering and formation of an extracellular matrix were apparently dictated by cell type, rather than by the alginate matrix. As indicated by the O'Driscoll scores, chondrocytes showed good cellularity, while BMP-4 cells and MSCs were moderate. This can be taken as evidence that the UHV/CG-alginate matrix maintains cell viability and that differences in cellularity must be traced back to specific features of the particular cell type. Recent experiments with encapsulated rat islets are in accordance with this view [26]. Formation of cell clusters could not unambiguously be correlated to cellularity. Transplants of BMP-4 cells exhibited the greatest number of clusters, whereas in transplants of chondrocytes and particularly of MSCs the occurrence of cell clusters was significantly less. In the modified O'Driscoll score cell cluster formation is considered negatively because such cell assemblies are not characteristic for healthy, normal articular cartilage or juvenile repair tissue [4, 15, 23]. In contrast, Wei et al. [34] and van Susante et al. [31] interpret cell cluster formation as a positive result, representing regeneration rather than degeneration. Therefore, the question remains open at present whether cluster formation is beneficial or detrimental to cartilage repair.

Formation of matrix proteins indicates that UHV/CG-alginate does not interfere with the secretory function of the encapsulated cells as was also recently demonstrated for encapsulated rat islets [26]. The level of type X collagen was quite low in the cell containing transplants (Table 1). Thus, hypertrophic chondrogenesis is not initiated by encapsulation in the UHV/CG-alginate matrix. Up-regulation of chondroitin-6-sulfate and chondroitin-4-sulfate was satisfactory and quite comparable for MSCs and chondrocytes, but not for transplanted BMP-4 cells. These cells produced only weak amounts of these 2 matrix proteins. Pronounced up-regulation of type II collagen was seen for encapsulated, transplanted chondrocytes and for encapsulated *in vitro* BMP-4 cells. MSCs exhibited also type II collagen expression, but less than type I collagen expression. Production of type I collagen was also observed for chondrocytes and BMP-4 cells kept in differentiation medium.

These findings suggest that re-differentiation of the cells upon encapsulation was subject to large (cell-specific) variations. De-differentiation under *in vivo* conditions apparently plays an important role in the case of BMP-4 cells because these cells were pre-differentiated *in vitro* before transplantation. In the case of chondrocytes and MSCs, however, other processes must be involved which trigger chondrogenic re-differentiation. It is well-known [8, 18, 24] that re-differentiation is influenced by a number of key factors: the physico-chemical properties of the 3D-matrix, low oxygen tension at the transplantation site and, crucially, the presence of appropriate growth factors. The nature and the detailed sequence of factors that are involved in the *in vivo* chondrogenic differentiation of mesenchymal progenitor cells are unknown to a large extent. So far, TGF-β-1 and IGF-1 were identified as important growth factors [16]. Lack of sufficient concentrations of these and other growth factors at the transplantation sites also seem to be responsible for the low chondrogenic potential of MSCs under *in vivo* conditions. In contrast to the BMP-4 cells, the MSCs transplanted in this study were not pre-differentiated *in vitro*. Thus, these cells relied solely on the supply of growth factors at the transplantation site. However, as shown by Schneider et al. [26] the alginate matrix can represent severe diffusion restrictions depending on the alginate concentration and the cross-linking procedure used.

Even though UHV/CG-alginate obviously meets important demands for clinical applications, it is essential to study the diffusion of growth factors in the alginate matrix and the associated re-differentiation steps under *in vitro* and *in vivo* conditions in more detail. Tools (e.g. the crystal gun) are now available to precisely match the permeability of the alginate matrix to the requirement for optimal, uniform diffusion of growth factors without detrimental effects on stability (see also [26]). Such work could pave the way for the use of MSCs and perhaps also for BMP-4 transfected cells in cartilage repair. Future work must also include detailed studies on the resorption processes of alginates under *in vivo* conditions once hyaline-like cartilage has been formed.

References

1. Ahrens M, Ankenbauer T, Schröder D, Hollnagel A, Mayer H, Gross G (1993) Expression of human bone morphogenetic proteins-2 or -4 in murine mesenchymal progenitor C3H10T1/2 cells induces differentiation into distinct mesenchymal cell lineages. DNA Cell Biol 12:871–880
2. Atala A, Cima LG, Kim W, Paige KT, Vacanti JP, Retik AB, Vacanti CA (1993) Injectable alginate seeded with chondrocytes as a potential treatment for vesicoureteral reflux. J Urol 150:745–747

3. Barry F, Boynton RE, Liu B, Murphy M (2001) Chondrogenic differentiation of mesenchymal stem cells from bone marrow: differentiation-dependent gene expression of matrix components. Exp Cell Res 268:189–200

4. Bentley G (1985) Articular cartilage changes in chondromalacia patellae. J Bone Joint Surg-Br 67:769–774

5. Binette F, McQuaid DP, Haudenschild DR, Yaeger PC, McPherson JM, Tubo R (1998) Expression of a stable articular cartilage phenotype without evidence of hypertrophy by adult human articular chondrocytes in vitro. J Orthop Res 16:207–216

6. Bonaventure J, Kadhom N, Cohen-Solal L, Ng KH, Bourguignon J, Lasselin C, Freisinger P (1994) Reexpression of cartilage-specific genes by dedifferentiated human articular chondrocytes cultured in alginate beads. Exp Cell Res 212:97–104

7. de Bernard B, Bianco P, Bonucci E et al. (1986) Biochemical and immunohistochemical evidence that cartilage an alkaline phosphatase is a Ca^{2+}-binding glycoprotein. J Cell Biol 103:1615–1623

8. Domm C, Fay J, Schünke M, Kurz B (2000) Die Redifferenzierung von dedifferenzierten Gelenkknorpelzellen in Alginatkultur. Einfluss von intermittierendem hydrostatischen Druck und niedrigem Sauerstoffpartialdruck. Orthopäde 29:91–99

9. Dornish M, Kaplan D, Skaugrud O (2001) Standards and guidelines for biopolymers in tissue-engineered medical products: ASTM alginate and chitosan standard guides. American Society for Testing and Materials. Ann N Y Acad Sci 944:388–397

10. Gibson UE, Heid CA, Williams PM (1996) A novel method for real time quantitative RT-PCR. Genome Res 6:995–1001

11. Häuselmann HJ, Masuda K, Hunziker EB, Neidhart M, Mok SS, Michel BA, Thonar EJ (1996) Adult human chondrocytes cultured in alginate form a matrix similar to native human articular cartilage. Am J Physiol 271:C742–C752

12. Hierck BP, Iperen LV, Gittenberger-De Groot AC, Poelmann RE (1994) Modified indirect immunodetection allows study of murine tissue with mouse monoclonal antibodies. J Histochem Cytochem 42:1499–1502

13. Kergosien N, Sautier JM, Forest N (1998) Gene and protein expression during differentiation and matrix mineralization in a chondrocyte cell culture system. Calcif Tissue Int 62:114–121

14. Leinfelder U, Brunnenmeier F, Cramer H, Schiller J, Arnold K, Vásquez JA, Zimmermann U (2003) A highly sensitive cell assay for validation of purification regimes of alginates (submitted)

15. Marijnissen WJCM, van Osch GJVM, Aigner J, Verwoerd-Verhoef HL, Verhaar JAN (2000) Tissue-engineered cartilage using serially passaged articular chondrocytes. Chondrocytes in alginate, combined in vivo with a synthetic (E210) or biologic biodegradable carrier (DBM). Biomaterials 21:571–580

16. Nöth U, Tuli R, Osyczka AM, Danielson KG, Tuan RS (2002) In vitro engineered cartilage constructs produced by press-coating biodegradable polymer with human mesenchymal stem cells. Tissue Eng 8:131–144

17. O'Driscoll SW, Keeley FW, Salter RB (1986) The chondrogenic potential of free autogenous periosteal grafts for biological resurfacing of major full-thickness defects in joint surfaces under the influence of continuous passive motion. An experimental investigation in the rabbit. J Bone Joint Surg-A 68:1017–1035

18. O'Driscoll SW, Fitzsimmons JS, Commisso CN (1997) Role of oxygen tension during cartilage formation by periosteum. J Orthop Res 15:682–687

19. Paige KT, Cima LG, Yaremchuk MJ, Vacanti JP, Vacanti CA (1995) Injectable cartilage. Plast Reconstr Surg 96:1390–1398

20. Paige KT, Cima LG, Yaremchuk MJ, Schloo BL, Vacanti JP, Vacanti CA (1996) De novo cartilage generation using calcium alginate-chondrocyte constructs. Plast Reconstr Surg 97:168–178

21. Passaretti D, Silverman RP, Huang W, Kirchhoff CH, Ashiku S, Randolph MA, Yaremchuk MJ (2001) Cultured chondrocytes produce injectable tissue-engineered cartilage in hydrogel polymer. Tissue Eng 7:805–815

22. Peterson L, Minas T, Brittberg M, Nilsson A, Sjogren-Jansson E, Lindahl A (2000) Two- to 9-year outcome after autologous chondrocyte transplantation of the knee. Clin Orthop 374:212–234

23. Poole CA, Matsuoka A, Schofield JR (1991) Chondrons from articular cartilage. III. Morphologic changes in the cellular microenvironment of chondrons isolated from osteoarthritic cartilage. Arthritis Rheum 34:22–35
24. Rajpurohit R, Koch CJ, Tao Z, Teixeira CM, Shapiro IM (1996) Adaptation of chondrocytes to low oxygen tension: relationship between hypoxia and cellular metabolism. J Cell Physiol 168:424–432
25. Rudert M, Hirschmann F, Wirth CJ (1999) Wachstumsverhalten von Chondrozyten auf unterschiedlichen Trägersubstanzen. Orthopäde 28:68–75
26. Schneider S, Feilen P, Cramer H, Hillgärtner M, Brunnenmeier F, Zimmermann H, Zimmermann U (2003) Beneficial effects of human serum albumin on stability and functionality of alginate microcapsules fabricated in different ways (submitted)
27. Schuurman HJ, Hougen HP, Van Loveren H (1992) The rnu (rowett nude) and rnuN (nznu. New Zealand nude) rat: an update. ILAR News 34:3–12
28. Schwinzer R, Hedrich HJ, Wonigeit K (1989) T cell differentiation in athymic nude rats (rnu/rnu): demonstration of a distorted T cell subset structure by flow cytometry analysis. Eur J Immunol 19:1841–1847
29. Steinert A, Weber M, Dimmler A, Julius C, Schütze N, Nöth U, Cramer H, Eulert J, Zimmermann U, Hendrich C (2003) Chondrogenic differentiation of mesenchymal progenitor cells encapsulated in ultra-high-viscosity alginate (submitted)
30. Temenoff JS, Mikos AG (2000) Review: tissue engineering for regeneration of articular cartilage. Biomaterials 21:431–440
31. van Susante JL, Buma P, Schuman L, Homminga GN, van den Berg WB, Veth RP (1999) Resurfacing potential of heterologous chondrocytes suspended in fibrin glue in large full-thickness defects of femoral articular cartilage: an experimental study in the goat. Biomaterials 20:1167–1175
32. Walker GD, Fischer M, Gannon J, Thompson RC Jr, Oegema TR Jr (1995) Expression of type-X collagen in osteoarthritis. J Orthop Res 13:4–12
33. Weber M, Steinert A, Jork A, Dimmler A, Thürmer F, Schütze N, Hendrich C, Zimmermann U (2002) Formation of cartilage matrix proteins by BMP-transfected murine mesenchymal stem cells encapsulated in a novel class of alginates. Biomaterials 23:2003–2013
34. Wei X, Gao J, Messner K (1997) Maturation-dependent repair of untreated osteochondral defects in the rabbit knee joint. J Biomed Mater Res: 34:63–72
35. Zimmermann U, Hasse C, Rothmund M, Kühtreiber W (1999) Biocompatible encapsulation materials: fundamentals and application. In: Kühtreiber WM, Lanza RP, Chick WL (eds) Cell encapsulation technology and therapeutics. Birkhäuser, Boston, MA, pp40–52
36. Zimmermann, U, Mimietz S, Zimmermann H, Hillgärtner M, Schneider H, Ludwig J, Hasse C, Haase A, Rothmund M, Fuhr G (2000) Hydrogel-based non-autologous cell and tissue therapy. Biotechniques 29:564–581
37. Zimmermann U, Thürmer F, Jork A et al. (2001) A novel class of amitogenic alginate microcapsules for long-term immunoisolated transplantation. Ann NY Acad Sci 944:199–215
38. Zimmermann H, Hillgärtner M, Manz B et al. (2003) Fabrication of homogeneously crosslinked, functional alginate microcapsules validated by NMR-, CLSM- and AFM-imaging. Biomaterials (in press)

Future Perspectives

Skeletal Tissue Engineering in Cartilage Replacement: Future Perspectives and the New Age of Regenerative Medicine*

21

ROCKY S. TUAN

Introduction

Tissue engineering is an emerging research discipline which aims to utilize the principle of biology and engineering to develop functional tissue substitutes. This new scientific field is poised to bring the practice of medicine into a regenerative phase, with the recovery of form, structure, and function of tissues and organs as the goal. Tissue engineering as a discipline began as application of biomaterials for tissue repair, and judging from the rapid increase in the number of research papers in the scientific literature, it is among one of the most rapidly developing biomedical research areas.

Tissue engineering is a particularly attractive technology for the treatment of skeletal diseases, most of which involve tissue degeneration or failure to heal. Chondral defects, generated as a result of trauma and injury or degenerative joint diseases, such as osteoarthritis, represent some of the most challenging orthopaedic conditions in terms of natural tissue healing and repair. Due to its acellularity, articular cartilage, when damaged or injured, fails to elicit significant reparative activity. Clonal proliferation of articular chondrocytes is often seen, and results in the production of mechanically inferior fibrocartilage. Extensive degeneration of the articular surface eventually necessitates total joint arthroplasty.

Components of Tissue Engineering

Although different tissues have different architecture and composition, there are 3 fundamental components in successful tissue engineering. These are *cells, scaffold,* and *environment.*

* The author is grateful to members of his laboratory who have contributed toward the understanding of mesenchymal stem cells and their application in tissue engineering, particularly E.J. Caterson, Ulrich Nöth, Richard Tuli, Wan-ju Li, David Hall, Genevieve Boland, and Keith Danielson.

Cells

Both, differentiated cells and tissue progenitor cells are candidate cells for tissue engineering application. Differentiated cells have the advantage that they are already fully committed to and engaged in the specific cellular activities of the desired tissue. However, since by definition the need for engineered tissues implies a lack of the original tissue and its constituent cells, differentiated cells can only be obtained by harvesting from healthy donor site (with inherent donor site morbidity), followed by subsequent expansion in number by *in vitro* culture, which often results in cellular de-differentiation. This effect could be due to either the inability of the differentiated cells to maintain their phenotype *in vitro*, or their low rate of proliferation, thereby allowing contaminating fibroblast-like cells to replace them in culture. These difficulties may be avoided if progenitor cells are used, since they may be allowed to first proliferate to yield clinically significant cell number, and then induced to differentiate into the desired phenotypes under controlled conditions. The isolation and application of these progenitor cells, often referred to as mesenchymal stem cells (MSCs), will be discussed later.

Scaffold

The three-dimensional aspects of tissues, particularly those of the skeleton, require that target engineered tissues be produced with the appropriate shape and form. A biocompatible scaffold is generally used for this purpose. In essence, tissue engineering is "reverse tissue development", since the scaffold, an articifial one, is first assembled, and then the cells are seeded, whereas normal histogenesis results from differentiated cells producing a tissue-specific extracellular matrix in which the cells reside. Additional functions of the scaffold may include its bioactivation, such that the cells are not merely lodged in the matrix, but instead are exposed to an environment that is conducive for tissue regeneration. In short, an ideal tissue engineering scaffold should be biocompatible, bioresorbable and biodegradable upon tissue healing, highly porous to permit cell penetration and tissue impregnation, permeable for nutrient delivery and gas exchange, and adaptable for the mechanical environment. The scaffold should have a surface that is conducive to cell attachment and migration, and permit appropriate extracellular assembly and the transmittal of signaling molecules.

Environment

Optimal tissue engineering is crucially dependent on the local environment to initiate and/or maintain the functional cell/tissue type. Regardless of whether differentiated or progenitor cells are used, the environment plays a key role in the successful outcome of tissue engineering. In general, the environment consists of bioactive factors, including signaling molecules, the appropriate extracellular matrix, and, for skeletal tissues, a mechano-biologically active component, such as mechanical loading. For cartilage tissue engineering, the most commonly used bioactive factors are members of the transforming growth factor-β (TGF-β) superfamily. TGF-β members are secreted growth factors that act via interaction with specific membrane-bound receptors to activate signaling pathways mediated by the Smad family of signaling molecules, resulting in the regulation of specific gene expression events. These intracellular activities in turn modulate cellular interaction with TGF-β and with other growth factors, as well as with extracellular matrix components. Dynamic loading is often used to simulate the compressive environment of cartilage and to activate chondrocytes.

Articular Cartilage Injury and Degeneration

Damage to the articular cartilage may result from physical trauma, when the joint is compressed under heavy load, or when angular or shear forces are applied to the surface, or from the consequences of degenerative joint diseases, such as osteoarthritis. The consequences include pain, swelling, joint stiffness, and may ultimately lead to loss of mobility. Osteoarthritis commonly occurs in the hips, knees, and spine; also it often affects the finger joints, the joint at the base of the thumb, and the joint at the base of the big toe. Osteoarthritis affects almost 20 million men and women in the United States. The chance of developing osteoarthritis increases with age, with most people over 60 having some degree of the disease, affecting at least one joint. Because the adult articular cartilage does not repair itself, lesions or degenerations are more or less permanent, and there is therefore a need for engineering cartilage for articular cartilage resurfacing.

Current Methods for Articular Cartilage Resurfacing

The most commonly used method to approximate articular cartilage resurfacing, for focal chondral defects, is microfracture of the subchondral bone, thereby eliciting the production of a fibrocartilaginous tissue to refill the surface. However, because fibrocartilage is structurally inferior to the hyaline articular cartilage, lesions usually reappear, resulting in further damage of the articular surface.

Osteochondral autograft or mosaicplasty is one of the current surgical methods for cartilage [1] (Fig. 21.1A). This technique is analogous to a hair-plug transfer. The surgeon removes a small section of the patient's own cartilage along with the underlying bone plug. This is obtained from an area which does not participate in high loading. This bone and cartilage (hence osteochondral) local graft is then transferred to the defect where a receiving hole has been prepared. Obviously, there is a limit to the amount of tissue available for "harvesting". The typical site of harvest is at the margin of the femoral trochlea – if that area is involved with damage then this technique may not be possible.

A recently adopted method for articular cartilage resurfacing is Autologous Chondrocyte Implantation (ACI) [2] (Fig. 21.1B). This technique originated in Sweden about a decade ago and recently has gained acceptance at orthopaedic centers across the USA. A small amount of the patient's own articular cartilage is harvested and through cell culturing techniques the cell number is increased from a few hundred thousand to over 10 million cells. These prepared cells are then reimplanted in the knee to repair and resurface areas of cartilage loss.

(A) Mosaicplasty

Donor plugs

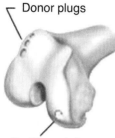

Cartilage defect
resurfaced with
donor plugs

(B) Autologous Chondrocyte Implantation

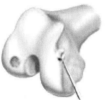

Chondrocyte
harvest

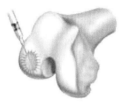

Chondrocyte
implantation

Fig. 21.1A,B. Current procedures for articular surface repair. (**A**) Mosaicplasty or osteochondral autograft, involving the harvesting and transplantation of osteochondral plugs; (**B**) Autologous chondrocyte implantation (ACI), involving the implantation of autologous chondrocytes into the chondral defect site under a periosteum flap.

While mosaicplasty and ACI have been effective in treating limited-size articular defects, donor site morbidity remains an issue of concern. There is therefore a need for tissue-engineered constructs that consist of cells that are derived from a non-articular cartilage site. Furthermore, it would be more preferable to generate implants that are not size-limited, such that large, non-focal defects may be repaired.

Cartilage Tissue Engineering

As stated above, successful cartilage engineering depends on the integration of cells, scaffold, and an environment conducive for cartilage tissue function. The following briefly outlines the current state of research along these directions.

Mesenchymal Stem Cells (MSC)

MSC are defined as adult tissue derived cells that exhibit the potential to differentiate into various mesenchymal lineage cell types, including chondrocytes, osteoblasts, adipocytes, fibroblasts, marrow stroma, and other tissues of mesenchymal origin. Interestingly, these MSC reside in a diverse host of tissues throughout the adult organism, and possess the ability to "regenerate" cell types specific for these tissues (Fig. 21.2). Examples of these tissues include adipose [3], periosteum [4, 5], synovial membrane [6], muscle [7], dermis [8], pericytes [9–11], blood [12], bone marrow [13], and most recently trabecular bone [14, 15]. Currently, bone marrow aspirate is considered to be the most accessible and enriched source of MSC, although trabecular bone may also be considered as an alternative source in view of recent findings of effi-

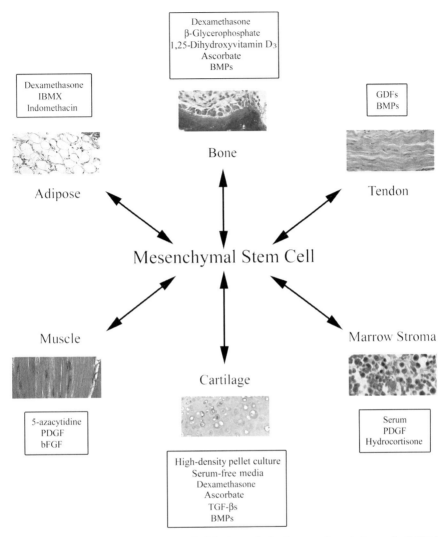

Fig. 21.2. Multilineage differentiation of adult tissue-derived mesenchymal stem cells (MSCs). This diagram depicts the *in vitro* differentiation potential of MSC *in vitro*, and some of the culture conditions necessary for directing the respective differentiation pathways.

cient multipotential cell isolation from this tissue [16]. Given the wide distribution of the sources of MSCs, the bone marrow stroma is likely to be the source of a common pool of multipotent cells that gain access to various tissues via the circulation, subsequently adopting characteristics that meet the requirements of maintenance and repair of a specific tissue type. In fact, the presence of MSCs in tissues other than the marrow stroma strongly suggests the existence of cell populations with more limited capacity for differentiation; specifically, mono- or bi-potent cells may have differentiation potentials developmentally adapted to (and perhaps restricted to) the tissues in which they reside.

Bone marrow contains 3 main cell types: endothelial cells, hematopoietic stem cells, and stromal cells. In a ground-breaking study, Friedenstein et al. [17] isolated cells termed colony forming unit-fibroblasts (CFU-F) from whole bone marrow, and showed that they were capable of forming bone and cartilage-like colonies. Many subsequent studies have substantiated the multipotent mesenchymal progenitor nature of cells isolated according to Friedenstein's method [e.g. 17–19]. These studies have prompted interest not only in the differentiation potential of MSCs, but also in the mechanisms governing their lineage specific differentiation, particularly to bone and cartilage. For example, Pittenger et al. [13] demonstrated that cells isolated from human marrow aspirates were capable of remaining in a stable undifferentiated state when cultured long-term *in vitro*, and that colonies derived from single isolated cells could be induced to differentiate along osteogenic, adipogenic, and chondrogenic lineages when provided the appropriate cues. Growth factors that have been used include platelet-derived growth factor (PDGF), transforming growth factor-β (TGF-β), basic fibroblast growth factor (bFGF), and epidermal growth factor (EGF), when MSCs are cultured in serum containing medium [20]. Current techniques for the isolation and *in vitro* culture expansion of bone-marrow derived MSCs range from aspiration and density gradient centrifugation to simple direct plating methods to size sieving [21, 22].

MSCs are described as multipotent cells owing to their ability, even as clonally isolated cells, to exhibit the potential for differentiation into a variety of different cell/tissue lineages (see Fig. 21.2). However, in most studies, it remains to be determined whether true stem cells are present, or whether the population is instead a diverse mixture of lineage specific progenitors. Inconsistency in the literature on the growth characteristics and differentiation potential of MSCs underscores the need for a functional definition of MSCs. At present, there is lack of a unifying definition as well as information on specific markers that define the cell types characterized as MSCs, with the sole definition being their ability to

- differentiate along specific mesenchymal lineages when induced to do so,
- remain in a quiescent undifferentiated state until provided the signal to divide asymmetrically, and finally,
- undergo many more replicative cycles than normal, fully differentiated cells.

Trabecular Bone Derived Human Mesenchymal Stem Cells

Our laboratory has recently reported the presence of multipotential MSCs in adult human trabecular bone [14, 16] (Fig. 21.3). These cells are isolated from bone chips derived from human femoral head specimens obtained after total hip arthroplasty. The bone chips are cultured in calcium-free medium, and cells migrate from the chips after 1 to 2 weeks of culture. These bone-derived cells proliferate for at least 25 population doublings with retention of multilineage differentiation potential. When cultured in appropriate medium under specific conditions, the bone-derived cells differentiate into osteoblasts, adipocytes, and chondrocytes. The requirements for chondrogenesis appear to be similar to those of bone marrow-derived MSC, i.e. the presence of TGF-β and culture at high density in a pellet. After 3 weeks in culture, the

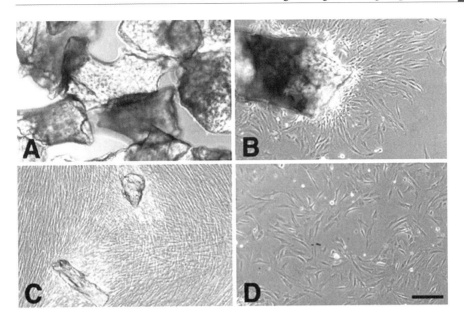

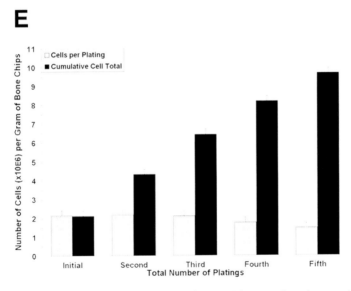

Fig. 21.3A–E. Adult trabecular bone derived multipotential mesenchymal progenitor cells. (A–D) Derivation of cells from bone fragments obtained from human femoral head after total hip arthroplasty. (A) Appearance of human trabecular bone fragments after collagenase treatment. (B) After approximately 10 to 14 days in low calcium-medium cells began to migrate from the bone fragments. (C) Cell cultures reached confluency after approximately 3 to 4 weeks in low calcium-medium. (D) Appearance of the first passage of cells harvested at 70% to 80% confluency from the bone fragments and plated as monolayer cell cultures. Bar = 200 μm. E MSC cell yields per gram of bone chips for a total of five consecutive platings of the bone chips.

TGF-β treated cell pellets display a cartilaginous histology, with alcian blue staining, and a fibrous collagenous matrix consisting of collagen type II. Compared to untreated controls, the TGF-β treated pellets are significantly larger in size and the extensive matrix formation is highly evident. We have recently developed a simple, high-yield procedure for the isolation of mesenchymal progenitor cells from human trabecular bone, using a reaming method of isolating bone chips, that require minimal culture expansion [16]. After four weeks, cells derived from the reamed bone explant cultures approached 80% confluence totaling 2.2×10^6 cells per gram of wet bone fragments. Interestingly, upon successive subculture of the bone fragments, obtained by curetting as described previously [14], a significant decrease in cell production was seen $(0.7 \times 10^6$ cells per gram) in the second plating, and by the third plating, cellular output completely tapered off with 0.07×10^6 cells per gram after an additional 4 weeks of culture. In comparison, cell yields per gram of reamed trabecular bone fragments were consistently maintained through four consecutive 4 week platings, diminishing slightly to 1.5×10^6 cells per gram following the fifth plating. The total number of cells generated per gram of reamed bone (9.7×10^6) following 5 successive platings of the bone chips was more than 3 times greater than that generated from chips obtained by the previous method of curretting $(2.93 \times 10^6 \pm 0.189 \times 10^6$ cells per gram). Moreover, these cells retain their ability to differentiate along multiple mesenchymal lineages through successive sub-culturing.

Ex Vivo Skeletal Tissue Engineering Using Mesenchymal Stem Cells

In addition to tissue-specific, differentiated cells, there are two undifferentiated cell types that may be considered for *ex vivo* tissue engineering: mesenchymal stem cells (MSCs), and mesenchymal progenitor cells. Stem cells are defined as cells that have extensive proliferative or self-renewal potential, and possess the ability to differentiate into multiple cell lineages. Progenitor cells, on the other hand, have variable propagation potential, and are committed to specific differentiation potential(s). A characteristic of both cell types is their ability to differentiate into a specific phenotype under specified conditions. Given their multipotential characteristics, MSC are generally preferred for tissue applications, since MSCs may also serve as a source for mesenchymal progenitor cells. *Ex vivo*, MSC-based tissue engineering has the following practical advantages:
- feasibility of obtaining a large number of MSCs;
- efficient expansion of MSCs without loss of differentiation potential; and
- controlled and defined conditions for tissue histogenesis, with or without scaffold materials, to produce tissues amenable for surgical implantation.

Crucial to the success of *ex vivo* tissue engineering is the ability of the tissue implant to integrate fully and functionally with the host tissues. Optimizing these properties is the goal of modern tissue engineering.

Cartilage tissue engineering has become one of the most active areas of tissue engineering, in view of the potential market needs and the scientific challenge of generating a three-dimensional, pressure-bearing tissue structure. Provided below are some of the recent and current research findings from our laboratory.

In Vitro Engineered Cartilage Constructs Produced by Coating Biodegradable Polymer with Human MSCs

We have recently reported the development of an *in vitro* engineered cartilage construct consisting of biodegradable polymer coated with bone marrow-derived human MSCs applicable for the repair of cartilage defects [23]. The construct was fabricated by press-coating a D,D-L,L-polylactic acid polymer block of 1×0.5×0.5 cm onto a high-density pellet MSC culture consisting of $1.5×10^6$ cells (Fig. 21.4). Following attachment of the cells to the polymer surface, chondrogenesis was induced by culturing the construct for 3 weeks in a serum-free chemically defined, chondrogenic differentiation medium supplemented with ITS-plus, dexamethasone, ascorbate, sodium pyruvate, proline and TGF-β1. The coated MSCs formed a homogeneous cell layer composed of morphologically distinct, chondrocyte-like cells, surrounded by a fibrous, sulfated proteoglycan-rich extracellular matrix. Collagen type II and cartilage proteoglycan link protein were detected immunohistochemically. Expression of the cartilage marker genes, collagen types II, IX, X, and XI, and aggrecan, was detected by reverse transcriptase-polymerase chain reaction. Scanning electron microscopy and histology revealed organized and spatially distinct zones of cells within the cell-polymer construct, with the superficial layer resembling compact hyaline cartilage. The fabrication method of coating polymer surfaces with MSCs allows the *in vitro* production of cartilage-polymer constructs of different sizes and shapes, which may be applicable as a prototype for the reconstruction of partial or full-thickness cartilage defects.

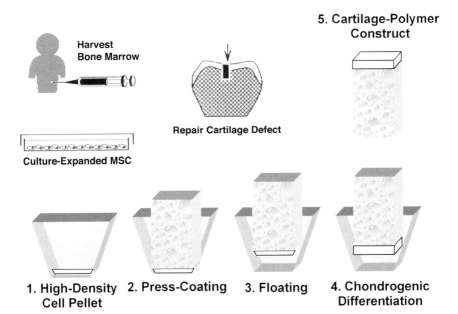

Fig. 21.4. Schematic of the fabrication of cartilage construct by press-coating chondrogenic MSCs onto a poly-L-lactide plug. Possible application of such tissue engineered cartilage construct for articular cartilage repair is indicated.

Three-Dimensional Cartilage Formation by MSCs Seeded in Polylactide/Alginate Amalgam

We have recently examined the potential of MSCs for cartilage tissue engineering by examining their chondrogenic properties within a three-dimensional amalgam scaffold consisting of the biodegradable polymer, poly-L-lactic acid alone, and with the polysaccharide gel, alginate. Cells were suspended either in alginate or medium and loaded into porous poly-L-lactic acid blocks. Alginate was used to improve cell loading and retention within the construct, whereas the poly-L-lactic acid polymeric scaffold provided appropriate mechanical support and stability to the composite culture. Cells seeded in the PLA/alginate amalgams and the plain poly-L-lactic acid constructs were treated with different concentrations of TGF-β1 either continuously (10 ng/mL), or only for the initial 3 days of culture (50 ng/mL). Chondrogenesis was assessed at weekly intervals with cultures maintained for up to 3 weeks. Histological and immunohistochemical analysis of the TGF-β1-treated poly-L-lactic acid/alginate amalgam and poly-L-lactic acid constructs showed development of a cartilaginous phenotype from day 7 to day 21, as demonstrated by co-localization of Alcian blue staining with collagen type II and cartilage proteoglycan link protein. Expression of cartilage-specific genes, including collagen types II and IX, and aggrecan, was detected in TGF-β1-treated cultures. The initiation and progression of chondrogenic differentiation within the polymeric macrostructure occurred with both continuous and the initial 3-day TGF-β1 treatment regimens, suggesting that key regulatory events of chondrogenesis take place during the early period of cell growth and proliferation. Scanning electron microscopy revealed abundant cells with a rounded morphology in the poly-L-lactic acid/alginate amalgam (Fig. 21.5). These findings suggest that the three-dimensional poly-L-lactic acid/alginate amalgam is a potential candidate bioactive scaffold for cartilage tissue engineering applications.

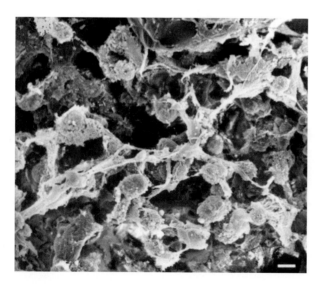

Fig. 21.5.
Scanning electron micro-scopic view of the morphology of MSCs seeded into alginate/poly-L-lactide amalgam and cultured for 3 weeks in the presence of TGF-β1. Note the presence of numerous round cells embedded in extracellular matrix, indicative of a chondrocytic phenotype. Bar = 10 μm.

Development of Nanofibrous Scaffold for Cartilage Tissue Engineering

Using an electro-spinning technology, we have recently successfully produced nanofibrous scaffolds using biodegradable polymers, including poly-L-lactic acid and poly (ε-caprolactone) [24] (Fig. 21.6). These nanofibrous scaffolds have fiber diameters ranging from 300 to 700 nm and a 90% porosity. MSCs seeded onto these scaffolds adhere readily to the nanofibers and display prominent expression of a number of cartilage-associated matrix genes, including aggrecan, collagen types II, IX and XI. Enhanced sulfate incorporation, indicative of matrix sulfated proteoglycan synthesis, is also observed, compared to MSCs cultured on tissue culture substrate, or even seeded as high-density cell pellets. Current efforts are devoted to testing the ability of these three-dimensional constructs to repair experimentally produced full-thickness articular cartilage defects in animal models.

Future Prospects of Tissue Engineering

Although there is currently a great deal of excitement in tissue engineering as a viable and potentially highly effective approach in regenerative medicine, there are a number of considerations and hurdles to overcome for the successful development of a tissue engineering product to market. The 3 most important criteria are:

- safety;
- satisfactory biological and mechanical properties and outcomes; and
- cost-effectiveness.

Starting from the early 1990's, there has been considerable investment made in the field of tissue engineering. For example, spending by U.S. tissue engineering firms has

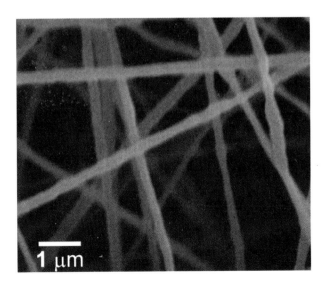

Fig. 21.6.
Scanning electron microscopic view of nanofibrous scaffold fabricated by electro-spinning of poly-(ε-caprolactone).
Bar = 1 μm.

increased almost three-fold since 1995 (US\$ 246 million in 1995, US\$ 675 million in 2002). On the other hand, at the same time, the value of publicly traded firms has dropped from US \$ 2.5 billion in 1995 to less than US\$ 0.5 billion. A great deal of uncertainty thus exists in the market place for tissue engineering product development. Added to this concern is the recent bankruptcy announcement of at least two tissue engineering-based companies. There are therefore serious challenges for tissue engineering from both the intellectual and the market perspectives. The intellectual challenges are clear, including identifying and optimizing usage of mesenchymal stem cells, fabricating of ideal scaffolds, developing functionality post-implantation, utilizing engineered tissues for the delivery of genes and gene products, establishing relevant experimental models, and developing off-the-shelf products. To meet these challenges, active and productive collaborations must take place between scientists, engineers, clinicians, governmental research and regulatory agencies, and device and biologics industries. At the market level, tissue engineering products must be scaleable, reproducible, safe for end-user, cost-effective, and be able to provide at least a reasonable alternative for current technologies. In parallel to the scientific and product development issues, a great deal of attention must also be paid to develop effective education programs for all the stakeholders in the tissue engineering field, particularly the patients, who ultimately must be convinced that tissue engineering products truly represent an improved treatment regimen that will restore function in an effective manner. Tissue engineering stands on an exciting biomedical threshold that will successfully usher in the field of regenerative medicine.

References

1. Bosch P, Musgrave DS, Lee JY et al. (2000) Osteoprogenitor cells within skeletal muscle. J Orthop Res 18:933–944
2. Brighton CT, Lorich DG, Kupcha R, Reilly TM, Jones AR, Woodbury RA 2nd (1992) The pericyte as a possible osteoblast progenitor cell. Clin Orthop 275:287–299
3. Brittberg M, Lindhal A, Nilsson A, Ohlsson C, Isaksson O, Peterson L (1994) Treatment of deep cartilage defects in the knee with autologous chondrocyte transplantation. N Engl J Med 331:889–895
4. Caterson EJ, Nesti LJ, Danielson KG, Tuan RS (2002) Human marrow-derived mesenchymal progenitor cells: isolation, culture expansion, and analysis of differentiation. Mol Biotechnol 20:245–256
5. De Bari C, Dell'Accio F, Luyten FP (2001) Human periosteum-derived cells maintain phenotypic stability and chondrogenic potential throughout expansion regardless of donor age. Arthritis Rheum 44:85–95
6. De Bari C, Dell'Accio F, Tylzanowski P, Luyten FP (2001) Multipotent mesenchymal stem cells from adult human synovial membrane. Arthritis Rheum 44:1928–1942
7. Diefenderfer DL, Brighton CT (2000) Microvascular pericytes express aggrecan message which is regulated by BMP-2. Biochem Biophys Res Commun 269:172–178
8. Friedenstein AJ, Chailakhyan RK, Gerasimov UV (1987) Bone marrow osteogenic stem cells: in vitro cultivation and transplantation in diffusion chambers. Cell Tissue Kinet 20:263–272
9. Hangody L, Feczko P, bartha L, Bodo G, Kish G: Mosaicplasty for the treatment of articular defects of the knee and ankle. Clin Orthop 391 [Suppl]:S328–s336
10. Hung SC, Chen NJ, Hsieh SL, Li H, Ma HL, Lo WH (2002) Isolation and characterization of size-sieved stem cells from human bone marrow. Stem Cells 20:249–258

11. Keating A, Horsfall W, Hawley RG, Toneguzzo F (1990) Effect of different promoters on expression of genes introduced into hematopoietic and marrow stromal cells by electroporation. Exp Hematol 18:99–102
12. Kuznetsov SA, Friedenstein AJ, Robey PG (1997) Factors required for bone marrow stromal fibroblast colony formation in vitro. Br J Haematol 97:561–570
13. Li WJ, Laurencin CT, Caterson EJ, Tuan RS, Ko FK (2002) Electrospun nanofibrous structure: a novel scaffold for tissue engineering. J Biomed Mater Res 60:613–621
14. Nakahara H, Goldberg VM, Caplan AI (1991) Culture-expanded human periosteal-derived cells exhibit osteochondral potential in vivo. J Orthop Res 9:465–476
15. Nöth U, Osyczka AM, Tuli R, Hickok NJ, Danielson KG, Tuan RS (2002) Multilineage mesenchymal differentiation potential of human trabecular bone-derived cells. J Orthop Res 20:1060–1069
16. Nöth U, Tuli R, Osyczka AM, Danielson KG, Tuan RS (2002) In vitro engineered cartilage constructs produced by press-coating biodegradable polymer with human mesenchymal stem cells. Tissue Eng 8:131–144
17. Osyczka AM, Noth U, Danielson KG, Tuan RS (2002) Different osteochondral potential of clonal cell lines derived from adult human trabecular bone. Ann N Y Acad Sci 961:73–77
18. Pittenger MF, Mackay AM, Beck SC et al. (1999) Multilineage potential of adult human mesenchymal stem cells. Science 284:143–147
19. Reilly TM, Seldes R, Luchetti W, Brighton CT (1998) Similarities in the phenotypic expression of pericytes and bone cells. Clin Orthop 346:95–103
20. Tuli R, Seghatoleslami MR, Tuli S, Wang ML, Hozack WJ, Manner PA, Danielson KG, Tuan RS (2002) A simple, high-yield method for obtaining multipotential mesenchymal progenitor cells from trabecular bone. Mol Biotechnol 23:37–49
21. Wakitani S, Saito T, Caplan AI (1995) Myogenic cells derived from rat bone marrow mesenchymal stem cells exposed to 5-azacytidine. Muscle Nerve 18:1417–1426
22. Young HE, Steele TA, Bray RA et al. (2001) Human reserve pluripotent mesenchymal stem cells are present in the connective tissues of skeletal muscle and dermis derived from fetal, adult, and geriatric donors. Anat Rec 264:51–62
23. Zuk PA, Zhu M, Mizuno H et al. (2001) Multilineage cells from human adipose tissue: implications for cell-based therapies. Tissue Eng 7:211–228
24. Zvaifler NJ, Marinova-Mutafchieva L, Adams G, Edwards CJ, Moss J, Burger JA, Maini RN (2000) Mesenchymal precursor cells in the blood of normal individuals. Arthritis Res 2:477–488

Subject Index

Printing: Druckhaus Berlin-Mitte
Binding: Buchbinderei Stein & Lehmann, Berlin